Praise for Finding True North

'*Finding True North* reminds me why I would rather consult a physician who at times struggles herself, rather than one who has remained above the fray, and how helpful it is to find the right place. In this case, Orkney. This is a story of struggling adults who find that True North is a place in oneself that is sustained by love and loyalty. We need a right place, and in the end we find and sustain True North in and for ourselves.'

Andrew Greig, author of
At the Loch of the Green Corrie

'An illuminating and enlightening book, beautifully illustrating the importance of place on our mental and physical wellbeing.'
Raynor Wynn, author of *The Salt Path*

'A quietly moving account of living with long-term depression that weaves together Linda's experiences as a doctor and a patient. With contemporary lifestyles that seem to be ever on the move, this book is a timely reminder of the stabilising effects of attachment to place.'　　　　**Sue Stuart-Smith**, author of
The Well Gardened Mind

'Linda Gask's writing and wisdom about depression are like no one else's and I turn to it time and time again to feel the comforting chime of shared experience.'
James Withey, author of *The Recovery Letters*

'Linda Gask is an experienced clinical and academic psychiatrist. She also suffers from depression and loves the Orkneys. It would need a master storyteller to weave these themes together into an intriguing, poignant and highly readable narrative. Fortunately, that is exactly what she is.'

Sir Simon Wessely, Regius Professor of Psychiatry,
King's College London

'This is recovery not as a political stick with which to beat the disenfranchised, but self-help and self-care that is truly transformative.' **Andre Tomlin**, Mental Elf

'Finding True North is beautifully written, in language that powerfully evokes not only the healing environments Linda has discovered in her quest. This is a memoir, but quite exceptional as Linda Gask brings not only her experience as a patient but also her knowledge, experience, and academic credibility as a leading psychiatrist. In no way sugar coated, it describes the struggles she has experienced in gritty detail but nevertheless offers hope. It is powerful and moving and quite exceptional.'

Kate Lovett, Dean of the Royal College of Psychiatrists.

'Deceptively easy to read given the deeper meanings being exposed, each new paragraph draws you on.'

Prof Tony Kendrick MD FRCGP FRCPsych (hon) FHEA,
Professor of Primary Care, Primary Care & Population
Sciences

'I really enjoyed reading *Finding True North*, especially the sensitive, thoughtful and informed discussion about the meaning of "Recovery".' **Professor Wendy Burn**,
President, Royal Society of Psychiatrists.

'Part novel, part journey of self-discovery and identity, this book offers the reader new insights into the most common mental illness, depression, reaching far beyond the academic aspects or, indeed, the usual "self-help" advice offered in many publications.'

Clare Gerada, Co-Chair NHS Assembly,
Previous Past Chair of RCGP Council
Member of BMA, RCGP and GPC Council

Linda Gask trained in Medicine in Edinburgh and is Emerita Professor of Primary Care Psychiatry at the University of Manchester. Having worked as a consultant psychiatrist for many years she is now retired and lives on Orkney. She maintains a popular mental health blog, *Patching the Soul* (lindagask.com), and contributes to Twitter as a mental health influencer. She is the author of *The Other Side of Silence* (2015), which was featured on BBC Radio 4 *Woman's Hour* and serialised in the *Times Magazine*. In 2017 she was awarded the prestigious President's Medal by the Royal College of Psychiatrists.

Also by Linda Gask

The Other Side of Silence

FINDING TRUE NORTH

The Healing Power of Place

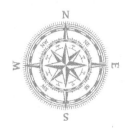

LINDA GASK

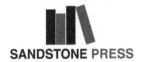

SANDSTONE PRESS

In memory of Maureen Johnston
– who welcomed me.

First published in Great Britain in 2021
Sandstone Press Ltd
Suite 1, Willow House
Stoneyfield Business Park
Inverness
IV2 7PA
Scotland

www.sandstonepress.com

Editor: Robert Davidson

ISBN: 978-1-913207-34-2
ISBNe: 978-1-913207-35-9

Sandstone Press is committed to a sustainable future. This book
is made from Forest Stewardship Council ® certified paper.

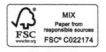

MIX
Paper from
responsible sources
FSC® C022174

Cover design by Stuart Brill
Typography by Iolaire Typography, Newtonmore
Printed in the UK by Severn, Gloucester

Contents

CHAPTER 1

A healthier life

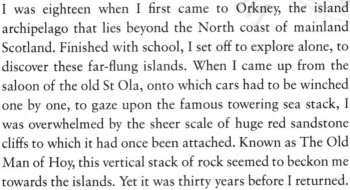

I was eighteen when I first came to Orkney, the island archipelago that lies beyond the North coast of mainland Scotland. Finished with school, I set off to explore alone, to discover these far-flung islands. When I came up from the saloon of the old St Ola, onto which cars had to be winched one by one, to gaze upon the famous towering sea stack, I was overwhelmed by the sheer scale of huge red sandstone cliffs to which it had once been attached. Known as The Old Man of Hoy, this vertical stack of rock seemed to beckon me towards the islands. Yet it was thirty years before I returned.

I've clambered through caves formed by hot springs in the heart of a glacier in the short summer of Iceland. Stared out to the ice floes of the grey-blue Baltic on the coast of Denmark. Whiled away the days on an agate strewn shore in North West Canada with the mountains of Alaska floating above the horizon. Walked on crisp snow in Arkangelsk in the middle of winter when the sun barely rises before it sets. For decades I was bewitched by the lonely beaches of the Western Isles of Scotland and held them in my mind as my spiritual place of retreat, an image of solace to call upon when times were hard. Yet I could never make a lasting home there. They would never be a place to which I would truly belong. I would always be a half Scots, but English speaking, outsider. Whether it was with the passage of time or a dawning realisation of the meaning of things, I finally acknowledged the need to return to Orkney. I have come here many times in the last decade to think, to write and, most of all, try to make sense of things. I now need to know if Orkney will be the place where I can patch up my life.

This morning I should be at my desk in the corner of the kitchen, by the front window of the house, but I am easily distracted. The fire in the stove has gone out. Beside the hearth is an Orkney chair with handwoven straw back, where I sit to read in the evening. A tall and narrow bookcase that holds what I'm currently working on is crammed into the corner next to the walnut writing desk that came with me from Yorkshire. A brass lamp lights the desk morning and evening; in the afternoon if there is sunshine my workplace is well-lit from the west. My pens and pencils are collected in an old mug decorated with the cover from Virginia Woolf's 'A Room of One's Own'. Of all the pots and pans packed to bring to Orkney, its handle was the only thing that the removal men broke in transit - hopefully it wasn't symbolic. Beyond the desk the latticed window, deeply recessed into the double layered stone walls of the old house, looks out onto a lawn and one rather stunted tree, surrounded by a patch of dense green wilderness that separates my land from the fields beyond. There are only a few houses scattered in the distance and no immediate neighbours other than wildlife.

One of those people who love nature but has forgotten the names of the animals and plants around them, I've been discovering my wild Orcadian garden. Some of the flowers are familiar from childhood: once carefully pressed between the pages of an exercise book for school. There's rather too much yarrow and rosebay willow herb, but in spring there are snowdrops, golden yellow crocuses, daffodils and a patch of bluebells nestled beneath the willow. Summer is a riot of wild pink roses as the rhubarb – ubiquitous in Orkney – begins to sprout, tart wild gooseberries appear and the clumps of montbretia by my desk window turn fiery orange. Then autumn arrives with a crop of berries from the tangle of brambles, the roses shed their petals and only bright red rose hips remain.

'There's a proper flower border somewhere under there,' Bob, who cuts the grass, told me last year.

'I'm not sure if I want you to hack it all back,' I replied. However, the rose bush has spread so much I feel like the sleeping beauty hidden from the world behind a forest of thorns.

It's a curiously still day, which means the squadron of flies which patrols the back of the house, in the lee of the breeze, will be out in force. It has been raining in the night and the flagstones are still wet. The sky is grey, but across the valley, behind the low hills I can see the purple mass of Hoy catching the sunlight from the East as it emerges from mist. The air is fresh and sweet, with only a hint of the farmyard smells of a couple of days ago, when my neighbour over the way decided to start muck-spreading. I made the mistake of hanging out my bed linen on the line, only to have to launder it again. Daffodils are coming out, and yesterday I saw new-born lambs in the field up the road. A blackbird is hopping about on the lawn and there are sparrows perched in the tree, possibly contemplating where in the eaves of my house to build their home this year.

I haven't spotted any hares in the last week.

'When you've been here a while, you'll start to see them everywhere,' my friend at the neighbouring farm told me the other day, but I haven't reached that point yet.

Last autumn, when the weather suddenly turned foul and a storm swept in from the Atlantic, I spied a young hare sheltering outside the back kitchen window, behind the house, crouched low with its long black-tipped ears resting on its back. I'd never been so close to a wild living thing, even if there was a double-glazed pane of glass between us. Every time I went to boil the kettle to make a mug of tea I said 'hello'. The hare trembled slightly as the wind ruffled her coat but studiously avoided eye contact. I'm sure she knew I was there. Rain and wind battered the house for three days, rattling the roof tiles and waking me in the middle of the night as it clanged the letterbox like an impatient visitor. When it eased off on the third morning the hare stood on all four legs, shook herself, lolloped gingerly to the corner of the garden and, a few moments later, was gone. I missed her company.

A psychiatrist, which is what I was for more than thirty years, is a medical doctor specializing in mental health conditions. I've helped many people to recover. I'm a Professor, an expert in my field, who has written numerous books and papers about mental health. However, all that knowledge has not made me any better at managing my own. That is still something I struggle with daily. Indeed, in my experience, the one question that health professionals rarely ask, but really ought to, must be: 'How do you get through the day?'

Those of us, like me, who are troubled by life problems and unresolved psychological conflicts have to find our own ways of living with our emotions. Many of us have 'residual' symptoms of depression and anxiety which wax and wane from when we get out of bed in the morning through hours of being, doing, feeling and interacting before getting back under the duvet. Surviving this daily experience is central to the process of recovery. I'm still working on the task of getting through the day on my own and adopting a healthier lifestyle.

Soon after I retired from work, three years ago, I set about finding a home here. I say 'I' even though I am married and have been for more than twenty years, but my husband John was still committed to a life in the South. There was a period after I finished working full time when I wasn't sure if I wouldn't be living here alone most of the time. We were staying together on holiday, only a mile away, when this cottage came up for sale. Described as a low white rendered cottage in the solicitor's particulars, it was situated in a shallow valley in the centre of the largest island of the Orkney archipelago, confusingly called the Mainland. It had an uneven flagstone path along the front and side and a lawn which looked as if it had been only recently fenced off from the neighbouring field.

It's not a traditional cottage. If it wasn't sturdily built the wind that blows from the west straight into the front door and my 'study' window would demolish it. My nearest neighbour lives in a new house with a windmill two fields away, and at each of the points of the compass there are tumbled collections of farm buildings to be seen in the distance. My friend lives at one of these, a quarter of a mile down the road. In the summer, her cows in the next field cluster around the fence with their calves, watching in fascination as I hang the washing on the line. In winter their bellows echo around the valley. There are few trees in Orkney and a scrub of willow is my only shield from the west wind. Cutting it back for the view may have been a mistake, but it was worth it to catch sight of the purple grey mass that is Hoy, the only really mountainous place on Orkney. If I cannot see water, I must be able to see a hill.

The house was built around the end of the nineteenth century as a but-and-ben, a simple Scots two room cottage, and was probably a farm hand's home as it stands on a plot at the corner of a field. Each generation of residents has extended it: a kitchen at the back, a loft room, and finally a wonderful airy lounge where the byre was once attached to a side wall. It was this room with its two front facing windows, a door opening directly into the garden and skylights through which huge shafts of sunlight split the soft warm air, that seduced me into buying. It took me almost a year to make it habitable, travelling up and down from Yorkshire.

Our basic physiological requirements are air, water, food, then clothing and shelter to protect from the elements: essential even for hares. It was winter when I took possession of the empty cottage, so I decided to fly from Manchester, limiting what I would carry. The first thing to arrive, a few hours after me, was a bed previously ordered from the local furniture shop. What I hadn't expected was for it to require 'self-assembly'.

'Is it OK for us to be off now?' the two young delivery men asked when they carried the last part of it into the empty bedroom.

'Yes, that's fine, thanks.' Too proud (and embarrassed) to admit to lacking practical skills I rushed off and purchased a screwdriver, as well as a kettle, tea and milk. Before the evening was out, I had at least warmed myself through and built somewhere to sleep, although there had been a few puzzling pieces left over that didn't seem to fit anywhere. The only effective heat was from an ancient coal stove in what had been the lounge, so that first winter was still Baltic despite the fire. I had to wrap myself in a duvet, night and day, as I used to when I was a student in freezing digs in Edinburgh. It did begin to feel as though I was trying to recreate my youth – but not in a good way – and I wondered if the whole proposition had been a mistake. The previous owners had decided they would prefer to live in Spain than Orkney, a decision I soon understood rather too well. My budget extended to fixing the heating, the kitchen and the bathroom, but getting the house waterproofed was more challenging. Facing west it gets the full blast of the horizontal rain that Scotland is famed for, the combination of gale force wind and water. Woken by a storm one night I stepped barefoot into a huge puddle of water that had been forced around the edges of the glass panes in the newly fitted front door.

'A porch – that's what you need,' the joiner told me.

'But won't the water simply soak the porch then?' I asked.

He shrugged. There's a price for living here.

Keeping my mind on track is essential as I am alone most of the time. It's a great place to practise the skills of allowing the boxes labelled 'difficult thoughts' to pass along the conveyor belt of my mind without having to unpack and ruminate over them. If I allow a worry to take over my mind here, it's quite difficult to elude it. My mood soon begins to spiral downwards.

Everyone's experience of what we call depression is different. For me, mood is paramount. Working and rushing around, I was probably less aware of it, yet my mood is a key part of my 'being in the world'. It's the lens through which I see what is happening around me, and its qualities colour, clarify or distort the ways I think about myself, the world and the future, much as the Hall of Mirrors in the seaside fairground where my father worked, warped reflections. Sometimes I was amused by the reflection; other times it horrified me. I've come to see that 'mood' is what must be managed if I am to reclaim my life.

The Surprise summit in the Peak District near my southern home is well-named as it rewards you with an unexpected panoramic view of the valley and peaks beyond. The crest of Howe Road near Stromness in Orkney usually has a similar impact because of the sudden realisation, as you top the hill, of a perfect composition. Here before you is the settlement nestled around the bay, framed by sea and hills, with the Hamnavoe ferry, when in dock, as its focal point. When John was in Orkney to celebrate his birthday a little over a year ago, that picture postcard view held no joy for me. As we drove down towards the harbour, the snow-capped island of Hoy rose from the sea to the west with the small island of Graemsay in front, with its two tiny white lighthouses which must be aligned by the captain of a ship to find the safe channel. It was a typically Scottish winter day, of the kind that reminds you how many different shades of grey there are between black and white. Sunlight tried to squeeze between the clouds with little success and the scarce winter daylight in Orkney echoed the approaching darkness inside me. I should have been relaxed, yet I wasn't. Everything positive about the day was ruthlessly filtered out by my mood. On the outside I could just about hold a smile, but inside I was barely holding myself together. The problem is that when I'm going down, I don't recognise it until quite late. Others see it first.

John put it succinctly. 'When you aren't well you start to talk all the time, and about 80 per cent of it is rubbish ... and you're doing that now.'

'I'm not, am I?'

'Yes, you are.'

What he was referring to is the emotional and verbal expression of anxiety, the constant seeking of reassurance and rumination on life's problems; the wringing out of my brain rather than my hands, in a way that drives those around me crazy. I've tried to learn my 'early warning signs' and the most obvious is the pain when my gut twists. I wander around drinking tea to distract myself and, in the past, have sent emails in the early hours only to regret them the following day.

John was right, I was becoming unwell again. The terrible feeling that there was a weight bearing down on my chest had returned, and I was exhausted and weary with the world. I stopped caring about my appearance and instead focused on the anguish and torment of what others couldn't see: feelings of guilt and despair and a terrible sensation of being *beyond* feeling, that the joy had gone out of being alive and there was no point to anything. The world had subtly changed from a place with potential for happiness to one I saw only in monochrome colours, one that seemed empty, hopeless or even dead, and attempts to change were doomed to fail.

There is a moment I recall from years ago when we first moved to Yorkshire. From the brow of the hill we saw the parish church in its centuries old position. If I had been of a mind to, I could have seen that the sky was blue with fluffy white clouds gliding past in the breeze and that the river Don was sparkling in the winter sun as it rushed towards Sheffield. Yet what I focused on that day was the dirty brown discoloration of the water at it washed over discarded beer cans, and the stench of the pollution from traffic as it poured through the village at the end of the pass. Thoughts rushed through my mind so quickly it was hard to grasp one for a closer look. A familiar sense that something terrible was going to happen and nothing could prevent it overwhelmed me. The professional side of my brain, watching from the sidelines, calls this Generalised Anxiety. The evil controller of my mind who is always there, waits to press the buttons marked 'churning of the stomach', 'trembling hands', or 'nameless fear'. The beauty all around me passed by and all I noticed were the blemishes.

A few days later we walked the same route, stopping for a moment to watch the river, and the world looked quite different. 'The level is lower than it was the other day and look! Spring is really here,' I pointed to an expanse of delicate white buds, a bed of snowdrops on the bank ahead of us, 'and the daffodils are coming up in the front garden too.' The rubbish and pollution were still there but were much less important. I was feeling positive about the world again.

'You didn't notice any of it the other day.' John sounded relieved. 'Before, you were preoccupied with how dreadful it was.'

The problems were still there but had receded into the background as they always do.

Mood is more than simply 'feelings' or 'emotion'. It's a longer lasting state of mind that encompasses all thinking. It can transform how events are viewed and change yesterday's great opportunity into tomorrow's disaster in the making. We aren't always aware of our mood but the people around us often are.

My boss for many years, a professor in the university, had a notoriously changeable mood. 'Be careful what you ask him about today,' his secretary, would warn me when I waited in silence outside his office, 'He's really grumpy.'

As I entered the room, he would, at best, greet me with an air of irritation, telling me with a grimace, 'Whatever you want, I doubt I can help you.' Other times it might be, 'Go away and come back when you've something useful to say.'

But then another day the atmosphere would be quite different, and everyone would know. The secretaries in the outer office would be chatting away, basking in the glow of good humour emanating from within. He would put his head around the door and call, 'Come in, come in, what can I do for you? Sit down and tell me all about it.'

Mood is not only the spectacles we wear but the overcoat we show to the outside world. Our mood is both us and yet *not* us. I cannot manage without my glasses although I know, rationally, that if I could will myself to change them the world wouldn't look as bad. Tomorrow, things may appear differently through them: brighter, sparkling and full of hope. When we're feeling positive, even the most boring things can seem worth doing. Mood balances on a knife edge and can change within the space of a few hours, but then it can remain stable for months.

Another problem for me is the 'timekeeper' with his stopwatch sitting somewhere in my head, usually insisting on what should be achieved each hour of the day. This is something I often observed in my patients. I don't set myself a raft of impossible goals on paper any more, although I have done. Revising for my final examinations at university, my obsessional planning got out of control to such an extent that I spent more time revising the plan than the knowledge. That timekeeper still measures out my day, and if I don't start something at the beginning of an hour, it can be difficult to start until another hour is up. I get stuck. I've lived with this problem all my life, and I know I'm not alone in this, but now I'm more aware. The danger is in counting away the hours of our lives.

Writing here, now, lifting my head every so often to watch the clouds scud across the sky outside my window, my mood is bright. It's much easier to be alone now than when I have been severely depressed. Last year, during a very low ebb, there was a period when I would spend hours waiting to get out of bed, only to feel so exhausted that nothing meaningful or productive was possible. Even reading a book was beyond me. To simply keep going, and not give up hope, I make myself set a few simple goals to maintain a daily routine: getting out of bed, washing, eating, eventually venturing outside for a walk.

'I feel so guilty about you taking care of me all the time

when you have enough to cope with already,' I would say to John, trying not to blame myself and descend further into a spiral of guilt.

My psychiatrist thinks, because it is clearly stated at the top of every letter he writes to my GP, who sends me a copy, that I have a recurrent depressive illness. Almost every word of that last sentence is contested.

Everyone has opinions on mental health and illness: 'experts' who have studied it; people who have experienced it and are called 'experts by experience'; those who have never suffered from it or know anyone who has, yet still have strong views. They all seem to know what you should do to 'get better' and 'recover', which generally means returning to your 'old' self. Many do, though some, like me, have persisting symptoms or relapse from time to time.

They wouldn't dream of offering advice to a heart attack survivor or someone with a broken leg. They don't understand that what they call 'depression' may only be the unhappy feelings they can usually shake off. So ... you can do that too. Yes?

This year I intended to get into a healthy daily routine here in Orkney, but don't get the idea that I am a virtuous paragon of self-care. I'm far from it. There is so much information about the kind of lifestyle I should lead but keeping it up gets harder and harder. It has to become a way of living, different from doing something for a limited period in the knowledge that your mood will improve. The fact is that I am going to have to change my lifestyle to reduce the risk of another relapse.

Yesterday I was good.

I got out of bed before 8.00 a.m., took my tablets for mood, blood pressure and thyroid, and ate a healthy breakfast. Ten minutes on the rowing machine in the attic and fifteen meditating (there is no point trying this any earlier as I find the sound of my breathing curiously soporific), left me with enough enthusiasm to do a few household chores and write for a couple of hours. After a lunch of soup and fruit I drove to Stromness for the shopping and walked to a seat overlooking the harbour, my favourite place in town. It bears a dedication to George Mackay Brown, who lived and worked in Stromness for his entire life, and who experienced long periods of depression. His former home is nearby, an unassuming council maisonette. Drawing on the inspiration of this place, the harbour with the hill called Brinkie's Brae rising behind, he created some of Scotland's finest poetry and prose, all rooted in the culture of Orkney.

With such a wide view I can see everything that is going on in my world. Weather permitting, I sit watching fishing boats come and go on the sapphire water: a person 'wild swimming' offshore; the Hamnavoe appearing from the west side of Hoy gradually growing in size as it comes into Scapa Flow, the great natural harbour between the islands. It's a roll-on roll-off these days, huge in comparison to the old St Ola. I would have gone for a longer walk but couldn't find the energy.

Back at home, I did some more writing and ate a fishy salad with lashings of olive oil, the closest you can get to good mood food in the north of Scotland. I drank no alcohol.

John and I talk on Skype most nights. I told him about my progress. 'I'm pleased you're getting exercise,' he said, 'but you could probably do with more than that.'

'So how did you spend your day?' I asked. He was in Yorkshire at the time.

'I walked up the hill behind the house this afternoon, then into the village and back. I spent half an hour on the exercise bike later.'

'Very good, that will help your blood pressure.'

'Tomorrow I've got to go over to Mum's for a couple of days.' His voice tailed off as energy drained out of him. I knew this visit would *not* be good for his blood pressure.

John looks after his mother who is suffering from dementia, caring for her not quite full-time but about half of the days of each interminable week and sometimes more. When I am back in Yorkshire, he is either at her house, exhausted on his return, or anxious and despairing about going back. John's elderly parents were the reasons we have stayed in Yorkshire for so long. His father died a few years ago, and his mother is alone.

'How can I help?' I have asked him so many times. 'How can I make it easier for you?'

'Stay well and take care of yourself properly,' he always replies.

She is in her late eighties, widowed but determined to stay in her own home and that her children will take care of her there. Since John was made redundant from his job as an accountant last year, and for a long period before, while he was coping with a demanding job, this has been his life and ours. He will not let me share the physical burden, but I try to help with the emotional one.

'Never mind,' he said. 'It won't be long before we're together and then we can do some walking.'

Inside I silently groaned. It is always wonderful to have

him here for a break, but he is so much fitter than I am. I find myself stifling something that might be frustration or even anger as I trail behind him. His stride is longer than mine, so he always ends up two steps ahead of his 'dutiful' wife.

There are advantages to living alone. I don't always have to behave well.

Indeed, why do I have to be good at all? I find it impossible to be good all the time. Can anyone truthfully manage that? Getting out of bed with a surfeit of energy and a full reservoir of self-control, I might keep it going for a few days but no longer.

Trying to lose weight, each day of the last week I have avoided cake, but today I gave in to a heavenly slice of apple tart with a scoop of ice-cream. Late out of bed, I couldn't be bothered with my morning exercises and got distracted by Twitter. I cannot keep up good behaviour indefinitely and then begins a vicious cycle because it is even harder to get going next day.

Western culture sets great store by self-discipline as a way of managing our fears, emotions and behaviour at home and in the workplace. If we cannot 'pull ourselves together' we must be weak. Trying to control ourselves we can make matters worse and undue attention to self-discipline can generate even more problems: have you ever tried to will yourself into sleep? Over-controlling becomes the problem even if the surprising thing is that self-control works as well as it does. Sometimes we can exercise it but at other times it's impossible. The pounds have disappeared in the past when I've been depressed, but when well, or taking certain pills, it takes a Herculean effort to lose them.

'I've been diagnosed with diabetes now on top of everything else,' I remember one of my patients, David, telling me. He had been feeling suicidal after a series of failed relationships but was just able now to cope with everyday life. In his youth he had been a professional sportsman – very fit and healthy.

'I know you have gained quite a lot of weight . . . I'm afraid it's probably the medication . . .'

'And the cream cakes,' he laughed, 'I can't seem to resist them . . . but I don't want to risk changing anything. I'm so much better than I was before.'

I wondered if he was just trying to please me, not only by telling me he was recovering on the pills I was prescribing, but also by not blaming them for his gain in weight – even though they were undoubtedly contributing. 'Everything you are on will be increasing your appetite.'

At that time, I too was struggling with a similar problem, only for me it was caused by craving sugary drinks to quench thirst – a side effect of the lithium that my own psychiatrist had started me on.

However, one of the pills David was taking, I now know, is very likely to cause major weight gain, which can trigger diabetes. Ironically the makers organised a lunchtime lecture for the medical staff at our hospital on the topic of 'managing diabetes', accompanied by a generous Indian banquet. 'Take as much food away as you want,' the drug representative called after us as we left the room. 'There's plenty left.'

'So much for our own health,' my colleague muttered as he filled a second container, then paused to explain, 'This is for my wife.'

Everyone departed laden with boxes of delicious curry.

Pharmaceutical companies traditionally seduce doctors with a free lunch.

For those of us who are patients, it sometimes feels as if the only way you can please your doctors, and everyone else (and be seen to be 'good') is to demonstrate how hard you are working at getting well: taking the prescribed medication, exercising self-control, getting back to your 'old self'. Your duty is to those who care for you and rely on you. The need to discipline your mind and body can become the most significant thing in life. Yet there is more to praise about a person than weight, blood results and compliance with the medication.

Still a rebellious child inside, if left to my own devices I would eat only bread, cheese, red fruits (and cake!) and drink plenty of orange juice and tea. I lived on that for almost year with the occasional meal out, and I was fine – really. And I so dislike going to bed. Without John to get me there I would sit lost in my thoughts, reading, tweeting, surfing the net or watching the TV for hours. Once in bed I can't get up and I can lie in bed half the morning like a teenager. When I was nine years old my mother took me along to the doctor's surgery expecting the GP to advise her (and me) what should be a reasonable bedtime. I know she was disappointed by his response. 'She'll sleep when she's tired.'

When we got home, she told my father in an exasperated tone, 'Well, he was only a locum. What would he know?'

An American psychiatrist I met many years later suggested I may have had Oppositional Defiant Disorder. I retorted, 'No, I don't! I've just always been difficult.'

My mother certainly seemed to think so, but my father didn't share her views. He would let me stay up late sometimes.

Like the night we saw in the first Labour government in more than a decade when I was nine years old, and the night we watched Ken Loach's *Cathy Come Home* to the very end where Cathy and her husband are driven apart by their homelessness. Those evenings, one jubilant and the other sad, helped determine the person I am today. I desperately want a happy ending but learned early that dreams rarely come true. I've always had this strange feeling that I must make each day last as long as possible, but a part of me can't wait for the next to come.

When I discovered that I had a serious physical illness too, just after I retired, part of me declared she was going to work so hard at being healthy that she would keep the disease at bay ... but I cannot control it, that is not possible, and I do not want to replace one all-consuming way of living with another. I have irritable bowel syndrome. Almost certainly this is related to anxiety, and the Lithium I took for mood problems has knocked out my thyroid gland, so I take thyroxine every day. If I'm not taking enough, I slow down and put on weight.

In those last few years at work, I had a creeping suspicion that I wasn't paying enough attention to my body. I didn't smoke and had a reasonably healthy diet, but was overweight, drank alcohol over the healthy limit for a woman and rarely took exercise. I suspected that taking better care would help to manage the exhaustion that enveloped me every evening and at the weekends, when I slept during the afternoons. None of that stopped me abusing my body, and now she is getting her own back. Little by little I became a person with chronic physical health problems, one, two and more ... to add to the on-going instability of my mood.

After giving up my regular job I found myself half-awake in an operating theatre for the third time in two years. There was an odd familiarity about it from my younger days as a medical student. The smell of the antiseptic hand wash; the immodest gown; the paper thin, cold, smoothness of hospital sheets. I was having a cystoscopy, a rather unpleasant procedure in which they put a tube inside you and have a look at your bladder. One thing about being a doctor is that other medics you consult about your insides always want to show off how their investigative toys work, and they think that because of your qualification you will be keen to see your own insides too.

'Take a look here,' the surgeon demanded. 'That's the bladder wall.'

To my surprise and relief everything looked fine, smooth and pink. Although I wouldn't have known whether there was something interesting to see, I was quite prepared to take the surgeon's word. He turned to put up some pictures which were from that morning's scan and for a few moments there was complete silence apart from the clattering of the nurses preparing for the next case.

'It's not cancer or a stone that's been causing the blood in your urine, but there probably is still an infection there.'

'Nothing else to see as you came out of the bladder?' I had been revising my urogynaecology on the internet.

'It all looked fine but, actually, looking at the scans, I think you have polycystic kidneys.' He didn't sound particularly concerned, just satisfied to have made a diagnosis.

I struggled to remember what that meant and the significance of it. The trouble with being medically qualified is that people assume you have a degree of knowledge which, if you are not a GP or a specialist in that area you've probably put in a locked filing cabinet at the back of your mind never to be reopened; or you still access it occasionally but, in my case at least, the notes are nearly forty years old and browning around the edges.

Ultrasound on the same day suggested the presence of cysts in both kidneys and liver. The radiology report suggested that one kidney was enlarged. Or at least that was what the surgeon said. I couldn't make out anything from the image on the screen. 'You'll have to go and see the Renal people,' he said as the nurses wheeled me into the recovery room.

Only six words: 'I think you have polycystic kidneys,' but there is nothing simple about being given a diagnosis. It means interaction with a new world of people and initiation into a different way of life: doctors, nurses, therapists, surgeons, technicians, and the places you will find them, the new hospital clinic you haven't been to before, the x-ray department, the laboratory, each with their own perspective on your body and/or mind. It is about learning to speak in a different language, about your memories, ideas, worries and expectations. All the other things you will have to do in your life, or have done to you, that you have never experienced before or hoped you would never have to – and remembering all those other things that you intended to do, but now perhaps never will.

I didn't have much memory of how kidneys should work. Blood flows in and urine flows out. The kidney works magic between. The first patient whom I cared for long enough to get to know as a person, and whom I then saw die, had kidney disease.

Andrew's illness was very different from my own. He was in his thirties and had been diagnosed with diabetes in his adolescence. He came into hospital in Edinburgh after a viral illness sent his damaged kidneys into failure. I listened in the ward office to the team of doctors from the renal ward when they discussed his case.

'He is still quite a young man . . . ' one argued.

'But he already has serious vascular complications . . . partial blindness, some nerve damage, as well as his kidneys,' another responded.

'And they don't do well on dialysis you know,' the consultant concluded, 'we rarely take them.'

It's different now, people with diabetes receive dialysis and kidney transplants but back then we all understood that for Andrew this was a death sentence.

A few days later his health had deteriorated further despite our attempts to keep him alive. I watched from the door of his room when he said goodbye to his tearful wife and children. I felt even more helpless as she wept at the sheer unfairness of his so unexpected passing as the ward sister lead her into another room. 'Oh God no. No! Help me, please . . .'

Although feeling fitter than I had for years, I also felt as though my body had let me down. Something was happening over which I had no determination. After the surgeon delivered his verdict, I felt numb. Like many people, I spent hours online researching the subject until the rational part of my brain was exhausted. Collapsing onto the easy chair in my study I burst into tears, sobbing until my throat was hoarse, my chest tight, and my shirt wet with tears. John put his arms around me.

'I'm here,' he whispered. 'We'll get through this together, I can give you one of my kidneys.'

'It's not as easy as that.' I was overwhelmed by his love and willingness.

'I know, you have to be a match, but I've been reading it up too you know.' He tried to smile. 'There are things you can do, donating into a pool so that you can find someone who does match and swap with them.'

'I don't know if it will ever come to that. Anyway, I might be too old.'

'I am not giving up on you. Ever.'

By then I was grieving for the loss of my health, and the hopes I had for the future, and it all seemed so terribly unfair. Just when I had given up the work that was gradually killing me and was about to start the life I had postponed for so long, something else was going to do that anyway. Developing a chronic illness necessitates a fundamental re-thinking of one's biography and self-concept.[1] It certainly feels like my lifeline had been fractured and it is still physically painful. Life changes must be made to keep my blood pressure under control, which is crucial in chronic kidney disease.

Now I know and accept that I have had a genetic disorder for many years, and which is going to get worse as I get older, at a rate as yet undetermined, and may eventually need dialysis. I have a friend who is much older with the same diagnosis. She has avoided dialysis, but her brother was very severely affected and died in middle age.

As the nephrologist said to me when I first saw him, 'It is something you have always had. It isn't new. Its autosomal dominant so you have a 50 per cent chance of developing it if one of your parents carries the gene, but in about 10 per cent of cases it's a new mutation.'

He couldn't understand why investigations carried out in my early thirties hadn't revealed the problem. As the years passed, the timer on my kidneys has been ticking away silently and the cysts have been slowly growing in size, squashing the healthy tissues into destruction. Programmed into me at birth it was probably running quite slowly otherwise it would have been noticed much sooner and I might have had a transplant in my thirties.

Meanwhile, I carried on a lifestyle of overwork and emotional exhaustion. I didn't have to decide what to do to change my life, because I fooled myself that there wasn't a decision to be made. Yet, like so many of my patients, I suffered because I struggled not only to live what was increasingly an impossible existence but refused to admit how impossible it was.

'You cannot go on like this,' John said, many times, 'you are going to damage your health even more.'

How much he worried about me became etched ever more deeply into his face as the years went by. However, there have always been things that he doesn't understand, because he is quite different from me in at least one essential way. He is one of those people who can eat two cooked meals a day and not put on weight regardless of exercise.

As I sit here writing at my desk, occasionally looking out the window at the world beyond, a little voice inside shouts *but you have to look after yourself physically because of your kidney disease. You should exercise, keep your blood pressure down, work at it.* I know that is why he worries, but I cannot let his fears take over my life. I have enough of them myself.

Over the last few weeks a cat has visited the garden from time to time. She is pacing about on the windowsill in front of me now, framed by the lawn, the bushes that are beginning to bud and the purple hills beyond. She is hungry and knows I have food for her. The other evening, I drove the eleven miles to the supermarket to stock up for when she came to call. I take a saucer from the kitchen cupboard and open another tin for her.

'Are you going to come in? Come on.' I put the saucer inside the hallway, crouch down and reach towards her with one finger. Cats usually cannot resist butting a pointed finger and she moves towards it, but then backs off and will not come in. She stops at the threshold as though at an invisible force field. She desperately wants to eat but she is also fearful of coming too close, so I move the saucer onto the flagstones outside. Even though she is small, she is quite self-possessed and clearly her own feline. She will decide if she is ready to push our relationship a little further.

It's 4.00 in the afternoon. The wind is getting up again, and with it has come more rain. Clouds have darkened the sky even though it is still hours before sunset and the sofa beckons. The Controller is telling me I have had a useless day, that there is no point doing much else because the day is ruined. All afternoon I have been trying to stop my ruminative thoughts and telling myself each time the hour passes that I should somehow re-start the day and do something worthwhile. My mood has been spiralling downwards.

I call John on his mobile. It rings, and I leave a voicemail. A few minutes later he calls back. 'I'm just at the hospital now with Mum. Is everything OK?'

There sometimes comes a point when I cannot continue by myself. I hate to ask for help, but I need it. 'I just wanted to hear your voice. I miss you.' Yes, I do miss him. I know I am fine on my own most of the time, but not always.

'You sound a bit down.'

'I've done nothing today.'

'Great,' he says. 'I like to hear you are practising that. Now take the rest of the afternoon off. Watch a film. Read a book. Enjoy your retirement! I give you permission.'

I don't need him to say that, but when I am unable to say it to myself it can really help.

You would think that after all the therapy I have had in my life I might have taken the controller in my head to one side by now, punched him (I always think of him as male) in the face and told him to fuck off. Sometimes I can do just that. There are times when I can almost forget that he is still there and others when it feels like he will never leave me. Most of the time I am somewhere in between. I know that the need to be doing the 'right' thing is to do with seeking approval from others and is a very powerful driver. We can become very self-critical because of the way others have criticised us in childhood and that can lead to fear, anxiety and depression later in life. Along with these can come feelings of shame about what others think of us. Changing how we live our lives is hard, and recovery certainly cannot depend on achieving the 'gold star' of always doing the right thing. More likely it has to do with recognising that isn't always necessary. Our need for perfection in living a 'disciplined life' can sometimes be more to do with our inner controller than needing to please those around us by working at 'being healthy'.

I cannot help the feeling that time is passing increasingly

quickly, and the hours are getting fewer as I count them. I try to learn how to make every day seem a little longer and begin to work my way down what is left on my bucket list of life. I'm thinking of everything I wanted to do when I had enough time, everything and everyone I promised I would make space for when I returned to work. I always thought there would be a future time when I would be able to cope with life, but in Orkney my future has arrived. It is here, and now.

Sometimes I shelter from the storms of life for days on end, like the hare outside my kitchen window, keeping my head down until it seems safe to venture out again, concentrating on surviving and simply 'being'. At other times I may find something that energises those parts of my brain that 'being good' simply doesn't. Reading more than for years I am learning how to waste time. In some ways I am still approaching, and then retreating, from living the life I know that I could lead.

We all need a place where we can be ourselves. Here in Orkney I see my likeness in the landscape: deceptively bucolic with darker depths like the mysterious Neolithic stone circles, and angular edges where lush green fields roll over vertical precipices, high above a foaming sea. Simply being here is good for my health. My blood pressure is lower, and the longer I am here, the easier it becomes to accept failing to meet my targets. We make these targets for ourselves, so we can break them. We can listen to the advice of others but, ultimately, we have the freedom to choose our own goals and make our own decisions about how we want to live.

Two and a half years since I arrived, the Wee Hoose has become my place to retreat into from the world. The old wounds are beginning to heal, but some remain half-open, and there are times when I still feel vulnerable and at risk of further harm.

CHAPTER 2

Other people

Orkney can get very warm in July and August (warm for me anyway, I get burnt sitting next to a 40-watt light bulb), but it is almost always breezy, which keeps the midges away. John visited for a month but has gone back to Yorkshire. I am alone again. The cruising season is almost over, and it's a huge relief. Luxury liners call here through the summer and tourists are ferried from one place to the next seeing all the 'highlights' in a day, including the obligatory stop at a whisky distillery and the Standing Stones. Only here for a few minutes at most, they take selfies with Neolithic monoliths before putting both hands on them in hope of being transported to the eighteenth century, as in *Outlander*. Visitors rarely make it down the lane to the house, but the other evening I was disturbed by someone knocking at the door after eleven o' clock. A couple, who had spotted my lamp in the window, handed me a letter written in German and asked, in broken English, for directions to their bed and breakfast. After recovering from the shock of having late night callers, I managed to explain they had a few more miles to travel.

Today the Sands O' Wright in South Ronaldsay, the south-ernmost of Orkney's inhabited islands, are almost empty, and I take off my shoes and socks to tiptoe into a seascape that would not be out of place in the Mediterranean. With gentle waves glistening in the sunshine, the bay is confined at each end by rocks, leaving pools to explore at low water. As the depth changes nearer the sandy shore, colours trans-mute through shades of blue and aquamarine to sea green. A few wild swimmers brave the chilly water, but no-one else ventures forth just yet. Holding my breath, I step into the surf and soon acclimatise. This is my favourite beach even though it doesn't have the pristine, sweeping grandeur of the Western Isles, which is where I retreated in the past when times were tough. Pungent green and brown sinews of seaweed are strung along the tide line, and a couple of battered caravans look as though they have been abandoned to the elements, but this is the place where I can quite simply be me. Sometimes though, I avoid walking here, because being alone under the vast skies, without the distraction of music other than the wind and the sea, forces me to pay attention to what is happening inside.

The last time I was severely unwell, a year ago, I experienced anxiety unlike any before, much of it from interactions with 'other people'. My sinews felt tight as the strings of a harp stretched taut over my bones, vibrating every time they were roughly plucked. I could only tolerate company for short periods, and the effects persisted for hours. After retirement, I had carried on doing occasional work in Manchester. This meant going to meetings, which can be difficult for me at the best of times. One especially has lodged in my memory.

I knew everyone well. Some were old colleagues, from when I worked as a doctor with a particular organisation which I had helped to set up. However, that didn't prevent me thinking I would rather be anywhere than with them at that moment. They asked all the usual questions.

'How's Scotland then? Cold?'

'You must have a lot of snow.'

'What on earth do you find to do all the time. Don't you get lonely?'

'It's an island? Is there a shop to buy food?'

'Why did you want to go and live there anyway?'

I have my answers: 'It's actually warmer in Orkney than in Yorkshire at the moment. We are at sea level, so we don't get much snow. There are plenty of shops. We have three supermarkets. I went to university in Scotland and always wanted to return. I would love to be there right now!'

That day I couldn't get into the spirit of things. Listening mostly, I felt distant from the banter, even excluded.

After the meeting I drove into the city centre and walked into the huge Arndale Shopping Centre to buy things for my computer. In my first placement in psychiatry at the Royal Infirmary as a junior doctor, being able to walk around the centre was top of the hierarchy of anxiety-provoking situations that people experiencing severe agoraphobia had to master before being discharged, and I've always been fearful of not being able to find my way out. The 'avenues' all look the same with garish windows full of sparkly bling. I was sent from one electrical shop to another for the right piece of hardware and when I came out of the second, had no idea where I was. There was a sinking feeling in my stomach, my heart rate accelerated and I was suddenly soaked in perspiration. An assistant looked concerned and I managed to ask, 'Which way is out?' She pointed and I ran, gasping with relief in the cold air of the street.

Most people in England have little idea what life is like in Orkney. I rarely meet anyone who has visited, but that's fine with me (though it is getting harder to keep it a secret). I went to Manchester to train as a psychiatrist, and, although I have practised my trade in other Northern cities, I have been at the university as a student or academic for almost all the years since then. I am used to laughing off questions from those who cannot imagine leaving that city. I used to think that way. It was exciting for someone who came from the Lincolnshire coast, much more so than Sheffield, our nearest 'big city' and Edinburgh where I studied. I loved living in Manchester in my twenties and thirties. It is the place where I decided to leave my first husband whom I had married too young, to embrace a hedonistic lifestyle with the enthusiasm of someone who missed out on their adolescence whilst studying hard. Unprepared for adulthood, my survival was down not only to my therapist but also my mostly female colleagues, the nurses and social workers in the mental health team. The pubs we visited after work have disappeared now, but the memories remain.

Late one evening we were all on the sticky dance floor of the Continental Club when a couple of men tried to push in.

'Watch out, you could be sectioned if you're not careful,' shouted my friend Susan. 'We've got a psychiatrist (pointing to me), a social worker, and I'm a psychiatric nurse.' Wisely, they edged away.

That night there were more people crammed into my Mini than I have ever driven home, before or since.

Manchester, with its infectious capacity for rebellion and scientific invention – the atom was first split by Rutherford in a laboratory near where I worked – helped me to rediscover myself after my divorce. Now I barely last a couple of days there, and long for the peace of the country.

Some friends think John and I make an unlikely couple, and, in many ways, we are quite different. My cats selected him from all the other eligible men in our street in Manchester. However his politics, which the cats were less interested in than his willingness to feed them, are quite a bit to the right of mine. There was a period when he read the Guardian but, now, he is back with The Times (never the Telegraph). Despite tribal differences, our values are not very different. He is warm-hearted, soft, generous, loyal, and knows far too much about James Bond while I get excited about maps and timetables, but we share a dark sense of humour. We have both been married before and learned quite a few lessons the first time round. We never had children, only cats, and they are now all gone.

Last year, when I was feeling so anxious, alcohol was the only thing that could shift the tension. It took John's version of the *Casino Royale* 'Vesper', a lethal combination of gin and vodka, to calm me. Mindfulness exercises didn't touch it and exercise was difficult as I was exhausted most of the time. When the sun returned, the green shoots of the daffodils I had planted pushed through the grass verges behind our Yorkshire house. There is something particularly awful about feeling depressed as spring arrives. Suicide rates peak at these times, not in winter as might be expected. No-one understands why, but signs of renewal might heighten the contrast between the outer and inner worlds: one dark, without hope, and the other bathed in sunlight.

When people ask me to explain why some of us become depressed, I tend to draw on the concepts of vulnerability and stress. A combination of genetic factors, early life experiences and life stresses add to our vulnerability, such that, when a torrent of events comes along, those with the lowest thresholds get washed away while the more resilient remain standing.

Both of my parents experienced anxiety and I am pretty sure my father got depressed too, though he never had treatment. My middle brother has obsessive-compulsive disorder, which he developed as a child, yet the youngest seems unaffected by the family heritage of 'nerves'. I feel sure that genes are only part of the story – they get 'switched on and off' by things that happen to us in our environment and what happens early in life is crucial. I didn't suffer any major traumas, but my family was far from 'happy', and my severe episodes have always been triggered by life events, usually losses.

That time the trigger was grief, something I know about given my delay in grieving for my father who died in my early twenties. Grief is a normal response to loss but the power of grief for animal companions is often wrongly dismissed by those who fail to understand how important those attachments can be. My beloved cat Sophie went missing from our house in Yorkshire. I spent two weeks searching for her, walking all around the village calling her name, my heart rising at the slightest sign of grey tabby fur in the distance.

One morning I was heading home when an elderly lady who was walking a black Labrador called out to me. 'Are you looking for a cat?'

'Yes, a grey tabby. Have you seen one?'

'Rex found something a few days ago, in the woods up there.' She gestured up the lane, towards a place I knew Sophie loved to hunt. 'I took it off him. I can show you where we left it.'

My heart was thumping as I followed her to a stone wall next to some stables and peered over. Amongst the weeds there was something that looked very like the head of a cat.

'Do you think it's her?' the lady asked, sounding concerned. Her dog, possibly remembering where its bounty had been hidden, began to look interested.

'It... it could be. Thank you.' Rooted to the spot, I could neither look over the wall again or leave.

'Are you OK?' she asked, 'It must be a bit of a shock. It was last week. It wasn't my Rex who did it. He just found it.'

'I'm sure he didn't.'

She paused for a moment, and said, 'Goodbye, then ... Oh, I'm so sorry to give you such bad news!'

When John came home, we went back to the stables and he clambered over the wall. It was recognisably her, probably killed by a fox. We buried her in her favourite place in the garden, under soil warmed by the sun beneath the south facing lounge window.

If, when Sartre said, 'Hell is other people' he meant the perpetual struggle with the idea of how we are regarded by others, then that perfectly describes something that has troubled me for much of my life.

Many of us spend our lives paralysed by worry over what other people think, but I have learned to cope by creating a confident persona for myself, someone who can perform when out 'in public'. Allowing myself to become someone else is liberating but also very tiring because it's a performance, and I still fear those situations when I enter a roomful of people. Somehow, I am always the anxious individual standing in the corner with a glass of wine while pretending to look at the bookshelves. I have never acquired the skill of working a room.

Joe Moran talked in *Shrinking Violets* about how shyness can make us retreat from others, tongue-tied and blushing, but it can also make us seem quite the opposite – awkwardly loud and unable to stop talking – which he calls barking shyness. Been there!

As someone who has taught people how to communicate truthfully and directly about things that really matter, such as love, life and death, part of me has dismissed the inanities of everyday chat. So much time is wasted by people avoiding the important things they need to say to each other.

At a conference in Atlanta, Georgia, nearly twenty years ago, I approached two people who were talking over drinks. One of them has become a good friend and has probably never thought about it again. The man she was talking to replied sharply, 'Actually, we're having a private meeting here.'

I muttered something like, 'Oh my apologies,' and slunk off for another glass of wine.

Why this upset me so much I don't know. He would have probably said the same thing to anyone who tried to butt in, but I know I am too sensitive and thin-skinned and easily hurt.

When I've been severely depressed, paranoid notions have made me avoid other people even more. However, the other side of sensitivity is that, when functioning well, I am fairly tuned in to the feelings of others, which has helped me understand and empathise with patients. Moran tells how the psychiatrist, W.H. Rivers, who treated First World War soldiers suffering from shellshock, employed his shyness to help him face the world with a kind of gentle curiosity. A personal style, which his patients no doubt greatly benefited from. In my clinical work I was able to manage my shyness because the person was seeking my help and being the real me was an important element. My patients needed to be able to not only share their feelings with me but sometimes about me too, without fear this would damage our relationship.

Carol was a widowed ex-dancer in her early sixties who never failed to tell me what she thought about my appearance. In her youth she had travelled the world performing in exotic locations.

'Black nail polish. Black!' she exclaimed one afternoon, looking down at my hands, 'What on earth . . . I wouldn't be seen dead in that!'

'So, you don't approve? What would you suggest?'

'You want to know what I think?'

'Well I hope you can tell me,' I smiled. Usually I dressed all in black but perhaps the overall effect was a little too gothic and downbeat. When Carol's mood was high, she could, as her polite restraint melted away, ask quite personal questions of me, and make her feelings quite clear.

She once brought me a fridge magnet as a gift which stated, 'Never trust a doctor whose house plants have died,' which summed up the state of my office. However, though this conversation sounded on the surface like our usual banter, I sensed an undercurrent – it was also about me taking her opinions seriously. Always elegantly dressed, she had previously confided that her regular visit to me was one of the rare times she changed out of her dressing gown. I had told her then how honoured I felt.

Today, taking a deep breath, she told me firmly, 'Something brighter! If I can make an effort, then you can too!'

Genuineness of demeanour is crucial because, when you are seeking help for mental health problems, you can spend a great deal of time worrying about what the therapist thinks about you, rather than focusing on what they need to know. You filter out what you are too frightened, embarrassed or ashamed to talk about until you realise that you are re-enacting your most difficult encounters. Those painful moments when you were either confirmed in your fears or hopes about their motivations.

There's the rub for people like us, because who we become is ultimately determined by our relationships with significant others. The problem is that if we do not tell others how we are feeling no-one will be able to fathom our suffering. Unfortunately, some professionals make hasty judgments about what we need without sufficiently engaging us in meaningful conversation. They observe and interrogate us like an 'object' rather than treat us as an equal person.[2]

A little while ago someone I know, who like me has experienced mental health problems for years, told me how she can predict what questions her psychiatrist will ask. 'Usually he begins with "how has your mood been?" just as I sit down. Then it's "how are you sleeping?", "what is your appetite like?", "have you lost or gained weight?" "has there been any point when you've felt life isn't worth living?" And of course, "are you still taking all the tablets?"'

Our conversations with patients are so predictable. 'Do you ever feel able to say anything about how difficult life can be for you?' I asked, realising how fortunate I'd mostly been in my own experiences.

She looked at me with a quizzical expression – as though the answer was obvious. 'No, I don't. I don't think he really wants to know. He just wants me to say the right things and get out of the door.'

'Is that how it's always been?'

'Well there have been ones in past that seemed to want to get to know me as a person, but not now. I don't think they've got time.'

'I'm not sure it's only about time,' I said, 'although there's never enough of it.' But when we don't get to share our feelings, thoughts and fears with another person, we don't connect. It's little better than having someone walking around you, making notes on a clipboard while they glance at you occasionally. My shyness hasn't prevented me from recognising how important those connections are. If anything, the opposite is true. Building meaningful relationships where you can be honest with each other, and making them last, isn't easy.

As I walk along the beach today, I am aware of my mixed feelings about John's return to Yorkshire. Alone, I can focus on the things that are taking over from my work, the preoccupations that nourish my soul, writing in particular. Isolation forces me to practise things I know will help. When we are together, I don't get much writing done and feel guilty for losing myself in the laptop screen on my desk in the kitchen, rather than paying him sufficient attention. When he is alone, he is much more likely to catch the magical hour just before and after sunset which is the best time to take photographs. That can be very late in Orkney because, in in the white night of summer, when the days are endless, the sun almost never sets but seems to bounce slowly along the horizon like a pale balloon.

I've been with John for thirty years, and he has been the anchor of my life. Before therapy, and before I met him, I reached out for any kind of lifebuoy to cling to. Last night we spoke as usual at 10 o'clock.

'I'm looking forward to seeing you again,' I said.

'Me too,' he paused, 'even if there was a time a while ago when you wanted to live as far away from me as possible!'

'I reached a point,' I said, 'where I couldn't cope any more with you coming home each evening and finding fault ... with everything.'

'I know ... but I did take the hint, didn't I? It was a fairly big one too.'

We managed to laugh but I could tell from his voice that the hurt was still there. Our major difference is that John is the kind of perfectionist who likes his daily life to be in order, where I largely exist inside my own head.

We have been around this so many times. There have periods when it has been very hard work because both of us have found it difficult to cope with the stresses in our lives without taking it out on each other. I miss him terribly though. When I am alone my only physical intimacy is the kneading of a furry companion or the fingers of a masseuse, and neither compares with the joy of spooning in the morning with your loved one. Yet in the course of my life I've changed from a person who worried about being alone, to one who craves aloneness. I enjoy my own company but after a while I get lonely, and loneliness and depression are linked, especially as we get older.

Animals are important too, for providing us with emotional support when we have long term health problems, often with less associated stress than living with humans. Sadly, I am without feline company either.

The visiting grey tabby, whom I eventually named Katie (she shares Catherine Earnshaw's predilection for scratching plaintively on windows at night), has only returned once since the day I abused her trust. She had started to call regularly, hanging about the front lawn and rolling onto her back as though inviting a rub, but then running away when I tried. Anyone who has been owned by a cat will know that they usually want to be on both sides of the door at once. It seemed, for a while at least, that we knew exactly where we stood with each other and, besides, I was ambivalent about having another cat in my life when I wasn't here all the time.

At first, I thought she was a kitten, but her paws and ears were in proportion to her body, so she was simply tiny. When John saw her, he dismissed her as a 'scale model of a cat'. Possibly she had not been fed regularly or had worms. She also might be pregnant. So, my neighbour Pauline down the road, who has several cats of her own, brought up a trap and we lured her into it.

She stretched her lithe neck over the contact plate to reach the food but was unable to avoid putting a paw on it. The door slammed shut and she screeched with anger at the sheer injustice. Pauline repatriated her with her owners, who turned out to be at the farm across the valley. Katie didn't see this as in her best interest, but has only returned once since then, walking briskly through the garden, head held high.

I have been here by myself again for more than a month now. In John's absence (he knows the early warning signs only too well) I force myself to stand aside and do a quick self-appraisal. I'm mostly cheerful, getting a good night's sleep even though I need new blinds to shut out the white nights, and I have vivid dreams which I suspect are conjured by antidepressant medication along with dwelling on the past. I'm taking care of myself reasonably well, but without achieving the goal of preparing and cooking my own food. Feeling lonely I wonder about more therapy.

During my twenties and thirties, I underwent several years of psychodynamic therapy,[3] and freed parts of my personality I had been keeping under control. Sometimes the more assertive me who emerged was more of an abrupt and outspoken moth seeking the light of day, than a perfectly finished social butterfly. Nevertheless, it helped me address the difficulties I had in major relationships and take the risk of a second marriage. It helped me to live with myself, trust other people, and transform my story into one where the past wasn't constantly interfering with the present.

I developed strong feelings for each of my therapists (particularly the first with whom I undoubtedly fell in love) and began to understand how they were indeed emotions that were transferred from important people in my life. My first therapist was a man, with whom I began to deal with the unresolved grief I had for my father.

Dad and I had been very close in my early years. He had pushed me to do well, but when I won a place at a Grammar

School he became more distant. He didn't approve of my boyfriends or the way I dressed, or the fact that I had been altered by the middle-class culture he despised. His support helped me to become the class 'swot', which I also felt ambivalent about. It was an achievement, yes, but didn't do much for my self-esteem as a girl in a co-ed school where the boys only wanted to go out with girls doing Arts. There were very few of us who did science and, when we actually gained better marks, we became a threat to their self-esteem. In fourth year, when we chose 'O' level subjects, our little group of girl scientists, giggling across the Bunsen burners, were not viewed as suitable dancing partners at the school disco. There is an indelible memory of sitting along the side of the assembly hall, in my make-up and a new dress that I had taken so long to choose, a stylish (or at least I thought so) sixties tunic, with a zip all the way up the front, waiting for someone to come and ask me to dance, as those sitting with me were singled out and invited to stand up. Coming top of the class (physics and chemistry were considered to be masculine) did even less to improve my attractiveness to the opposite sex, and Dad seemed determined to keep it that way. Facial acne and having to wear NHS glasses for short sightedness hadn't helped either.

'You just need to focus on your education,' he told me. 'Nothing else really matters at the moment.' Except he was wrong. For an adolescent girl, her appearance and popularity can occupy a space in her head wildly out of proportion to their actual importance.

My first boyfriend had been a friend's older brother who hadn't attended our school so didn't know about my 'reputation'. One evening he came around to pick me up and Dad insisted I call him in. He immediately offered the bemused young man a drink, and then a cigarette. I exchanged glances with both. This was a game in which there was no right move. He would be damned if he accepted, and equally damned if he didn't.

Later that evening Dad handed down his verdict. 'A bit cocky if you ask me, barely hesitated.' He had been happier when I didn't have someone to go out with, but that was a lonelier place for me. When he died, we had grown a long way apart, pushed further by my competitive and jealous mother. Somehow it had been impossible for us to be close to him at the same time.

My first therapist tolerated my anger and ambivalence about the world and helped me to grieve for Dad, but I still have issues with powerful men and am acutely sensitive to rejection.

When I began to experience more severe and disabling episodes in my mid-thirties, I decided to try the tablets. I knew about the side effects but needed something to help me feel 'better'. There are times when engaging in any kind of talking therapy is difficult. Times when you can't get out of bed never mind make it to an appointment. Antidepressants got me to where I could use psychotherapy again.

Despite all this therapy, and taking tablets for best part of twenty five years, I tend to relapse every couple of years, ruminating constantly about my interactions: apparently simple things like telephoning a colleague at work or a conversation in the office kitchen. Did I say that the right way? What if they never want to speak to me again? I shouldn't have said that. What on earth was I thinking when I made that ridiculous joke? What did I tell them about that for – they will think

I'm shallow ... stupid ... showing off ... The list is endless, and I've managed them by seeking reassurances which haven't always worked. A downward spiral into depression follows.

That's why John is so attuned to an increasing frequency of rumination. It's a sign that things are not looking good.

Several years ago, I parked the car in a lay-by in the Pennines to call an old friend and colleague, seeking affirmation that we could continue to work together even though I found it difficult to cope with a key member of his team. In the distance smoke rose from a moor fire. The sight made me uneasy, remembering fires that had smouldered in the peat for months.

'I just wanted to know how things are? I'm sorry about how this has worked out,' I began. 'We've worked together well in the past. We can continue ... can't we?' Somehow, I knew that I couldn't trust that all would be well.

'Things have changed since we last talked,' he responded with an uncharacteristically cool tone. This other person had made a formal complaint about me, and something about his voice told me I was no longer worthy of his respect and friendship. My fears of rejection were realised.

Here was the evidence that I was shallow and stupid and offensive. I could feel the tears coming. It felt as if there was a crack in the snow globe that encapsulated my little universe and I was being sucked into the void by shame and guilt. Yet another part of me was saying: no, that's not right. Your assessment of things is correct ... your view of this world is valid and he has got it wrong ... keep trying to convince him. When my anger reached a crescendo he put down the phone. Within a few days my mood was much lower. I had been teetering on the edge of despair, ruminating over the problems in this relationship, and this was the final straw.

Today, as I sit on a rock at the Sands O' Wright, the sea reminds me of my father who only ever swam there, but it wasn't called wild swimming in those days. He never would trust swimming in a pool. At the memory of him a familiar knot of sadness rises but doesn't linger. Remembering him now with affection, I feel disappointment that he didn't live until we could deal with the problems between us as adults.

Children and dogs race in and out of the water and a little girl in a frilly bathing suit holds her father's hand as he wades out. She looks up at him, giggling, not yet having learned to be afraid. Wherever I have travelled in the world, I have dipped my toes in the sea in memory, but never learned to swim. I could never trust my father not to let go. Is it too late? Could I still learn?

Now I'm on an island to which I must sail. The author and psychiatrist Anthony Storr said we need time and space to discover what we are capable of. Being alone is a necessary step. When I was a child, I was often solitary, one of those introverted people for whom interacting with others without a break is a form of torture. Unfortunately, the world is full of extroverts who cannot understand and not all islands are solitary places. Once when staying on the Croatian island of Lopud in Mediterranean weather, I wandered over to another shore to escape the crowds only to find myself on a nudist beach. Escape from people, with or without clothes, was impossible. As an adult, I am re-learning how to 'be' with myself. I'm with Anneli Rufus who, in *Party of One,* complained how it's not easy to be a loner in a world obsessed with 'team-building', where the word 'loner' has connotations of being odd, crazy, secretive and strange. But it shouldn't.

A few years ago, while attending an international conference with several thousand others (my idea of hell), I spent a couple of evenings in a row with my Brazilian friend Sandra, and her group of colleagues. She asked me if I wanted to go out for a final dinner with them all on the last evening, but a quiet meal alone beckoned.

Sandra wasn't offended at my refusal, nor was she surprised. 'We are different. I need other people around me to relax and you need the opposite,' she laughed, hugging me. After too much time with other people, introverts need peace to allow the buzzing in our brains to quieten down.

Sadly, there is a real stigma to being on your own, which I suspect prevents some people embracing their solitude and learning to live with it. In my failing first marriage I knew more loneliness than when on a prolonged stay in a remote Highland cottage.

It can be tempting to spend more time in the company of others, to drown out your troublesome inner dialogue, but I wonder if I feel so at peace in my isolated stone cottage precisely because I am spending so much time on my own. Rarely with other people now, I avoid the problems of interaction. Is that healthy? Could my place of escape become an island prison? Perhaps I should make more attempts to join the island's thriving creative community which I am sure, if I am honest, would be good for my recovery. To find the level of interaction that is right. Not so much that it feels stressful, but enough to feel stimulated.

*

My final experience of therapy, Cognitive Behavioural Therapy (CBT), was anchored in the present, not the past. With it I learned more about how my mind works and discovered ways to challenge those ruminations. Previously unspoken, and difficult, 'Rules for Living'[4] were identified: strong beliefs that I should not criticise others; that I should live my life so that people will like me; my fear of relying on others. I still castigate myself for not being the person I should be. Attempting to live up to my high but conflicting standards led to anxiety. It is several years since that last course and I am beginning to realise just how long it can take for therapy to work. The skills must be continually practised.

Last weekend I visited my neighbour, Mary, whose cows have kept me under careful surveillance all summer. It was one of those late summer afternoons when the light is filtered through gold, and I walked up the lane and over the burn, revelling in the mild breeze coming from the South. Mary's family was visiting, and I wasn't sure whether I should stay. Like all the native Orcadians I have met she has always been very welcoming. I knew no-one in Orkney when I arrived here and met her as she was walking her dog up the lane. Every now and then she gives me some eggs from the hens that forage around her garden. On Saturday, her granddaughter, who was just learning to walk, was toddling between us all. Feeling guilty for interrupting their time together, I muttered, 'I should go and do something useful' and left, ruminating all the way down the road about whether I had implied that visiting her was a waste of my time.

Practising the techniques of cognitive therapy wasn't at all easy, but eventually worked. I didn't even have to seek reassurance from John on our call that evening.

It wasn't only a change in medication that got me throu the last time I was very low. First of all, I stopped pretendin to be well and accepted that I was feeling terrible: bleak, sad and empty. Paradoxically, this allowed me some leeway and it was easier to move forwards. I forced myself to keep going out even though I wanted to shut myself away and never come out again. I've met many people in my career who have done just that. Finally, I began to go out walking up the lane to the hill behind the house in Yorkshire. There is a superb view from the top of the moorland over towards the Pass, but in the decade we had lived there I hardly ever allowed myself the time, even though John walks it regularly. I did feel better afterwards.

Most of all, I was able to have an honest conversation with John about the uncertainty hanging over both of us. We had dreamed of living together in Scotland, but this had always been years away. Now it feels as though my future has arrived and I want to live it while I am still fit and healthy, but John still isn't ready to take that step.

'Two years,' he promised me. 'Let's look at things again then, how Mum is . . . I know you are worried about what is going to happen with your health, and I am too. But I need time, I need to care for my mother. It's different for you. You don't have those demands on you.'

My mother died a few years ago and we were pretty much estranged for a decade before. My middle brother Alan has severe mental health problems with which I tried to help in the past but spectacularly failed. Like me, and our father, he has his own way of being in the world, but he does now have support, which in the past he did not. My youngest brother Graeme is in the Army and we have barely seen each other

...e at eighteen to go to university. John's mother
...him to replace his late father in taking care of
...with her completely. From the photographs I
...looks exactly like his father did at the same age,
...of course he cannot replace him, and we have lives of our
own. Is it selfish of me to say that? Caring for others cannot
be at the expense of our own survival. We both need to hold
onto the hope that there will be a time when life will be easier.

I am not completely alone now, because of my relationship
with John, so perhaps that is why I find it easier to tolerate
my own company. I have many good friends, like Sandra, who
have supported me at difficult times over the last few years.
Not being a particularly sociable person, I don't have close
mates. My ideal is a person in the next room with whom to
have tea breaks and walks and share a bed, but I worry about
something happening to John before me, despite my kidney
disease and depression. However much I have declared my
independence, I do so love him, and have allowed myself to
accept his unselfish and tender care. We must be responsible
for ourselves and find ways to manage our difficult feelings
without causing pain to those we love. Precious relationships
can be damaged beyond repair with thoughtless words and
actions.

It's getting late and the breeze is getting stronger. Over to the
west the sun is sinking towards the horizon, but it will be a
few hours before it sets. Last night one of the farmers nearby
took advantage of the good weather, silhouetted against a
deep red sky as he brought in huge bales of hay with his
tractor. Later, in the blue hour after sunset, he continued
under lamplight until midnight, the sound of his engine

echoing across the valley. I climb into the car and drive the winding road back over the Churchill Barriers, causeways built by Italian prisoners of war. Whatever the reasons, they now make it possible for people to link up, communicate and work much more easily than before.

I came to Orkney because of a sense of community such as I have never felt anywhere else. It has starkly beautiful empty places, but also a welcoming population who never judge me for being an 'incomer' but instead invite me to get involved in whatever interests me, be it creative like the local writing group or caring, in the thriving voluntary groups. I'm just uncertain if I'm ready to do that yet.

My mobile just pings to tell me there is a message. There had been no signal at the beach. It's from Mary to confirm she'd love to go out for lunch sometime this week – I had left a message for her earlier. The only way I would ever know if I had caused offence was by trying to make contact once more. It's a kind of 'behavioural experiment'[5] and one worth trying. It cannot be worse if you expect to be rejected anyway. I am ridiculously pleased that she wants to see me again after all.

My car tyres crunch on the loose chippings of the lane as I drive back towards the cottage, past the ripening barley field rippling in the breeze. I am thinking about how life can be hard but how we come to terms with it, and the impact that has, is what living is all about. Other people may be part of the problem, but they are also part of the solution.

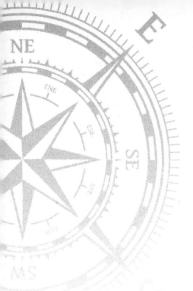

CHAPTER 3

Work

John drove back to Orkney with me for a holiday on the day before Christmas Eve. Within a few hours, an intense low pressure drifted with malevolent purpose across the North of Scotland, bringing storm force winds and driving rain under slate grey skies. The cold weather meant we had to light both stoves, the smaller in the kitchen near my desk, and the larger in the lounge. It was a miracle that the windows of the Wee Hoose stayed in place but the damp patch next to the window beyond my desk seemed to grow in size, and the recessed shelf beneath it swelled even more. The house needs attention, but nothing could be done before Spring.

Now though, Christmas is over.

'You are looking very tired,' says John. The bags beneath my eyes could hold a week's grocery shopping. I've crammed too much into the last three months.

'I mislaid my off button again,' I attempt to joke.

He smiles but I can see he is concerned. 'Let's get out of

the house today – we need to get some supplies in. You're not going to spend all day at that desk again.'

Work can be good for your mental health, but not always, and not any kind of work. Returning to work is often taken as an indication that you have recovered, but the reality can be different.

Two years ago, I took all the annual appraisals I'd accumulated over the years and slowly ripped up each sheet, determined that I would never consult again. If I had stayed in the National Health Service full-time and not moved to the university, I would have been forced into even earlier retirement. The British NHS proved not to be particularly sympathetic, either with my own episodes or that of my patients who worked in the system: doctors, nurses and allied professionals. The macho style of management made it difficult for people to return to work and was sometimes a key factor in a person becoming depressed in the first place.

One typically grey January morning in Manchester, I was back in the lecture room in the mental health unit at the Royal Infirmary to talk about my experience and understanding of depression, its causes and its treatment. Outside it was bitterly cold and flakes of snow were drifting gently past the windows.

When we tell the stories of our lives, we frame them in different ways – some helpful to others, and some less so. When someone has been ill, most people like to hear how they (sometimes 'heroically') struggled to a complete recovery. The person with cancer who has the all-clear at five years having been told that they were going to die long before then. The recipient of a heart transplant who goes on to live a full life for decades after. That is what others expect of us. To take the treatment and get better, or not take it and just 'pull yourself together and be fine'. For some of us it is more complicated. Our lives do not return to 'normal'.

The audience was a mixture of mental health professionals: doctors, nurses, social workers and psychologists and last, but not least, patients. The patients were not afraid to ask about antidepressant use and the latest treatments, because they didn't care about impressing with their questions – which many professionals do. Amongst the professionals some would have experienced depression for themselves but might not have reached the point where they could admit it or seek help. I had 'come out' and admitted it publicly, written about it, and told the truth. Nor was I ashamed. The story of my illness is a good one. I hoped they could listen and connect, and also take something away.

My experiences and those of my patients were often very much the same. In our complicated lives we had experienced loss, grieved, felt lonely, wanted to be loved, and sometimes self-medicated with alcohol. Some of us repeatedly made the same mistakes in our relationships. Many of us wanted, or had even tried, to end it all. I told them about my treatment: what helped, and what did not.

At the end, when everyone clapped, my anxiety returned. My hands were sweating, and the heart palpitations kicked back in. There were a couple of old colleagues and students there.

'You're looking well Linda! Retirement is doing you good.'

Yet, most of those who knew me best had not come. Perhaps they weren't interested because this wasn't a 'scientific' presentation, or they were embarrassed to hear another doctor talk about her own mental health. All these negative thoughts passed through my mind, but I dismissed them with a *maybe they are just too busy*, and the warmth of the audience contrasted with any kind of chilly harshness, either perceived or in the world outside.

As I was getting ready to leave, a young woman who had been sitting at the back approached. 'I'm a nurse,' she began. 'I've been really unwell, and it's so good to hear you talk about your own experience.'

'Thank you,' I replied, sensing she needed to say more.

'The problem for me is that I haven't recovered after just a few sessions of counselling – there's a lot in my past . . . ' she paused, 'The thing is, to have proper psychotherapy I have to come here, where I work.'

I understood that problem well. It's a thorny one. Yes, we shouldn't stigmatise mental health by hiding away, but the stigma of mental health problems exists even in mental health care. She would not want her colleagues to know she is receiving help and be fearful that someone might look at her records.

'I'm so sorry you are in that situation,' I replied, but there was nothing I could do to help. I really wished that I could.

There have been no boats in or out of the harbour for the last 24 hours because of the wild winter weather, and the shelves of the Co-op in Stromness are quite bare. The fruit and vegetable section could best be described as sparse, and there is no fresh bread. The icy wind has died down for the moment, so we walk up the deserted main street to my favourite viewpoint. The Hamnavoe is docked but a sign at the car park says there will be a sailing this evening.

'It's my parents' wedding anniversary today,' I tell John, breaking the silence. It's a companionable enough quietness but I have sensed that something isn't quite right. 'I was born ten months after the wedding and two weeks late. It had everyone counting on their fingers.'

We laugh, it's not the first time I've told this story. Probably not even the 21st but maybe there will come a time when each anecdote will seem fresh again. We just won't be able to remember what we had for breakfast. That's how it is now for John with his mother. She still watches *Coronation Street* but asks him to explain the plot to her every five minutes.

'I still think you are doing too much,' he says. This is what has been worrying him.

'I'm fine. It's nothing like it used to be.'

'Well, now it's a normal job, rather than double time. It looks as if you've got drawn into something that's getting you down. You always get pulled in ... Are you going to take on this new project you've just been offered?'

I've been asked to get involved in a review of mental health services in Orkney. It's something I really would like to do. 'I want to feel useful again,' I say apologetically.

'I know,' he says, 'but when will you have time for us?'

Later, sitting by the living room fire, surrounded by the tinsel and fairy lights that John took a day to put up, I say, 'The lights are amazing.'

'Look, they have several different programmes,' he replies. With the flick of a switch we progress through a performance of several different patterns of flashing.

He has also wound a short set of lights shaped like tiny spruce trees around the top of the headboard in the bedroom.

'I'm not sure how I feel about the flashing Christmas trees when I wake up, but I'm adapting.'

'It's good to see you smiling,' he tells me, 'We've spent so little time together since Dublin.' That was a couple of months ago. Even though I no longer consult with patients, I still do some training, and I was invited to Ireland for a workshop about depression, bringing the perspective of both a doctor and someone who has been in the other chair.

As we waited to board the plane to Dublin in Manchester airport, a group of women arrived wearing matching T shirts proclaiming they were the 'Girls on Tour' with a list of dates and destinations on their backs: 'Ibiza 2010', 'Amsterdam 2011' and so on. Two of their party sauntered away and a few minutes later returned with several glasses awkwardly balanced between their ultra-long fingernails. Something about their easy manner told me they worked together and were getting away from the daily slog to have a good time. In an odd kind of way, they reminded me of my mother. I could almost imagine her amongst that group because she enjoyed that kind of camaraderie and certainly wasn't shy. Meanwhile I was going to Dublin to work, to talk about mental health – a world away from the kind of work my mother did.

'I did all sorts of work as a student,' I whispered to John, 'but with those nails I could never have managed to do any of them.'

'Why on earth do you want to be a doctor?' asked my Scottish cousin who couldn't wait to leave school and find a job. I chose to go into medicine not only because it interested me, offered a step up in the world and the prospect of a regular income, but also provided a sense of self-worth and value beyond simply earning a living.

My parents both clocked in at 7.30 every morning and neither of them would have described their jobs as fulfilling. What they got was an opportunity to use their skills, a pay packet and the company of work colleagues. For my mother, for much of my childhood, that was with a group of women on a production line in a radio factory. My father preferred to be outdoors repairing rides in an amusement park. They never missed a day unless they were unable to get out of bed. No work meant statutory sick pay only.

As a student I cleared tables in cafes, worked on supermarket checkouts, served in a bar and waited on tables for employers who varied considerably in their attitudes to ill-health. Not best suited to waitressing, on more than one occasion I tipped a bowl of soup over a furious diner.

I was a much better barmaid. Standing up to drunks in a hotel in Ullapool who weren't happy about my refusal to serve them was good assertiveness training, and also provided me with insight into the nature of addiction. A local quietly said to me one day, 'If I ever ask you to put a double vodka in this tonic water you've just served me, please say no.'

He came in almost every day for the next few weeks. Then one day, as he sat at the bar with his glass, he looked up at me. 'Put a double vodka in this, will you, please.'

'You told me, a while ago, if you ever asked me to do that I was to refuse,' I replied.

He slid off the bar stool, left and never came back.

Meanwhile the hotelier, who would serve residents into the night before cashing up, began to accuse me of giving the wrong change – even though we bar staff all suspected his own state of inebriation every night was the cause of the errors in the till. I coped only because I could tell myself, 'This isn't what my life is always going to be like.'

However, it was the time I worked as an auxiliary nurse in Edinburgh, during the vacations, that provided me with the most powerful lessons about work. The women I worked alongside were miners' wives from the grey West Lothian coal mining villages who supported each other: laughing and joking when sharing smoking breaks in the cavernous bathroom at the end of the ward. Shedding tears when a patient they had cared for over many years died. Getting angry at something the ward sister had or hadn't told the visiting doctor about. Their husbands worked stripped to the waist and covered in coal dust, confined to spaces like the ones I would crawl through as a medical student trying to understand how miners developed lung disease (it wasn't difficult). From them I learned about the physical and emotional work of caring for older people near the end of their lives. Getting through the exhausting daily grind of catching the early bus each morning to the hospital. Washing, toileting, feeding, changing the beds and still finding time and energy for kindness.

'I have to do quite a bit of that now for Mum,' says John when I mention it, 'Sometimes it doesn't feel right, that I should be doing such . . . personal things for her.'

'But she wants you to do them and no-one else.'

'That's the really hard part.'

As untrained auxiliaries, now called 'healthcare assistants', we knew how difficult that work was. We spent more time than anyone else with the patients and could make a real difference to their lives, but our views were rarely listened to.

Alice was a tiny woman of about eighty years old, who spent her day curled into a ball in bed, her limbs stiff with contractures, with a large pressure sore on her left buttock which you could smell from the door of her room.

'Can't we get the doctor to look at this Sister?' we begged, 'Doesn't it need something else doing? Cleaning out? Packing?'

'No, we will just replace the dressing as before, and keep on.' Which we did ... until Alice died in pain from her own putrefaction. I didn't know enough then, being only early in my medical training, to challenge Sister's views, but I knew she had been wrong not to involve our visiting GP, and I can still feel the impotent sense of shame and anger that simmered amongst us on the day of Alice's death. I knew then that I wanted a job where I would not also become a powerless victim of the system in which I worked. That was the most important lesson for me.

'Those places are all gone,' I've said to John before now, 'It's all private nursing homes and care in the community.'

With elderly relatives he knows that only too well.

'You broke your tooth in Dublin last November,' John reminds me, as he throws another log on the fire. I'd had an argument with a crust of bread and ended up at the dentist. Like many young doctors working all hours, I didn't take adequate care of my teeth, and now I am paying the price.

No, that's not quite right, I didn't take care of myself at all, in body or in mind.

It had been several years since my last visit to Dublin. Then I had been lecturing to GPs about how to help people suffering from depression. Afterwards we all went for dinner and drank too much. I struck up conversation with someone with whom I'd previously had disagreements after he had defended one of my consultant predecessors against my criticism.

'You don't know what he had to put up with when he first arrived in that hospital, it was very tough.'

Our inhibitions loosened by alcohol we acknowledged we had both been trying to cope in an impossible environment. Mental health received much less attention than physical health care and our managers rarely sought the advice of doctors.

The day after arriving this time I faced a group of about thirty people, this time counsellors and therapists, who were waiting expectantly for me to talk about the same topic. 'Please excuse me if I'm not speaking as clearly as I should.' My audience were mostly women, as is usually the case, but they ranged in age from the very young to quite a bit older than me. 'Last night I broke a tooth.' There were expressions of concern. 'I've taken something for it and should be fine.' Somehow, I managed to keep going and there were plenty of questions.

'How did you cope with the stigma that there still is in our kind of work?' a young woman asked. 'What are your views about taking antidepressants at the same time as having therapy?' asked another.

At coffee time, I was approached by an older woman who wanted to talk about someone she had been seeing for a long time. Since I was no longer practising, I couldn't give her advice, but I could see that she needed to talk.

'I've known her for a year, and I am really worried about her. I just don't know what to do. It's keeping me awake at night.'

An older man started a conversation with me, while I washed down more painkillers with coffee. 'I still see the occasional client, but I've had to cut down. I was depressed too, and I went to see my GP'.

'Was it helpful?' I asked.

'She said, "Join the club!" I've seen a few doctors and nurses in my time for therapy ... ' He paused and looked directly at me. 'So, what do you think of all this resilience training everyone is asking about now?'

Not entirely sure what resilience is, I answered as best I could. Some people think it's an ability to remain well in the face of adversity. Others think it means you can 'bounce back' easily. Both our genes and what happens to us in childhood play a big part. Some people have a surfeit; others are more vulnerable. I am very sensitive to the ups and downs of life. I may have successfully survived a lifetime of work, but I've also had to use mental health services to keep afloat. I've not got through my career without serious wounds, but some people describe my survival as resilience. I call it bloody-mindedness.

'What can we offer to people?' he asked.

'I'm not convinced we can train them to be more resilient,' I replied, 'and it's not just a problem for the person, it's also to do with the environment they find themselves in.'

He agreed, 'I used to work in a company which was a very toxic place to be ... I know exactly what you mean.'

'I've worked in some of them too,' I told him.

Eleven years after finishing my medical training I finally became a consultant psychiatrist, at a time when the old asylums, which were built 'round the bend,' to keep them hidden from the world, were beginning to close.

Finding myself in charge of a ward in a huge Victorian mental hospital in Lancashire, I was horrified by some of the attitudes of the staff, whose families had worked there for generations. The building was decaying around us. Twenty years earlier there had been a scandal, and new brooms – including the psychiatrist I later criticised – had been brought in to sweep clean, but they too had become contaminated by the institutional malaise that Erving Goffman wrote so clearly about in *Asylums*.

'I gave evidence against a Chief Executive of a Mental Health Trust who was bullying female consultants who spoke up about things,' I said. 'Working in that hospital contributed to me becoming severely depressed.'

'What happened?'

'He left, as did the whole Board eventually, and I escaped to work for the University part-time in the end.'

My own GP supported me through that awful time. Another memory of Dublin is when I bumped into him at a conference there a few years later. 'You are looking much better,' he said, putting his arm around my shoulder and squeezing it, 'It's good to see you here.'

Every time we met in the surgery he would ask, 'How much longer are you going to stick out that job?' A couple of years after that chance meeting in Dublin and another severe bout of depression, I couldn't go on any longer.

'My Head of Department at the Uni said I was unmanageable too,' I smiled at the man who had asked my views about resilience. 'Actually, I took that as a compliment.'

I had the freedom to change direction, but a great many people with mental health problems are asked to return to work in conditions that are far from ideal. Low pay, no support and no sense of control, when it's very important for people with depression to have that feeling of being in charge.

Some of my patients had very negative experiences with their employers. One man was criticised for taking breaks to ensure he ate at regular times – he had Type 1 diabetes. When he got depressed again, they sacked him. Another young woman was a poster-girl for a 'back to work' scheme. The supermarket who took her on were keen to be involved but, after a few months, after the support from the hospital had been withdrawn and a 'success story' publicised, they expected her to 'work like everyone else'. The critical voices in her head returned and she became increasingly paranoid. She lost the job. In contrast, a patient of mine who worked for a large multinational was allowed to return gradually, over an extended period of time, and their occupational health department regularly called me to ensure I agreed with the plan. They did not want to lose such a valuable employee. Few other companies responded in a similar way.

Finishing the day by talking about the problems of working with caring professionals with mental health problems, I was reminded of a friend, a professor of Mental Health and former nurse, who wrote about how being depressed felt more stigmatising than the terminal cancer that finally took her life. Like so many of us, she found herself lacking when the talk turned to resilience. A terrible sense of guilt washed over me, for losing touch with her in the months before her death. Loss of people I care about is something I still cannot manage without avoidance, despite years of therapy, and I also tried to meet my own needs by being essential to others.

*

The world of my working life couldn't have contrasted more with the genteel squares of Dublin, with their multi-coloured Georgian doorways and iron railings, that we walked through on the way back to our hotel. Yet those ugly places where people struggle to survive are everywhere if you look closely.

In the few years before I retired from work, I returned to Salford, the city next door to Manchester, just across the River Irwell. Life is still hard there even in the twenty-first century. When people live in poverty, they are much more likely to experience mental health problems. Bad things happen to them more frequently in life and they don't have the resources to keep them afloat.

I had first been there as a young psychiatrist learning about child mental health problems. A social worker and I were visiting a young single parent living on the 9th floor of a tower block – one of several that still surround the run-down shopping precinct. She had just moved back to live with her own parents after the breakdown of her relationship, and her former partner was in prison. As she opened the door, we were greeted by her six-year-old daughter, a pretty little girl who danced towards us, twirling around in circles. She continued to twirl around and around and around the over-crowded space, completely absorbed in her own world.

According to her mother she spent much of her day performing this unearthly dance or screaming loudly every time she was prevented from moving. She had no language. I could see how much her mother and grandparents loved her, but their faces were lined with desperation. The young mother already had the air, and appearance, of someone at least a decade older than her years, something I came to recognise as a sign of inner-city hardship.

'I've been told she's autistic,' she said, starting to cry, 'but I don't know how to cope with her here … I just can't. I'm broke and next door keep complaining about the noise.'

Years later, I visited the same block with a young psychologist from our team to see one of her patients who was severely depressed and housebound. While we were talking with the young man in his lounge, a neighbour called by.

'This is the psychiatrist who's come to see me,' he told her, turning to us to say, 'She's a good friend, we all look out for each other here.'

'Psychiatrist!' she exclaimed. 'We could do with a resident here. When can you move in?'

I once managed to get a couple in their sixties rehoused from the top of a tower block to a terraced council house with a small garden. 'I can see the world again,' the lady thanked me. 'I was so depressed. I felt so cut off from people, it was so lonely only being able to see the sky when I sat in my armchair.' We don't spend our lives, when we are older, standing up to look out of the windows.

Successes like that were few and far between but made such a difference.

When I was down in London to give a talk about preventing suicide, a woman with a very Home Counties accent told me, 'Salford? I'd never heard of it until the BBC moved there!' I should have replied, 'I'm surprised because Marx and Engels knew it well,' but I didn't.

John gets up to put some more coal on the dying fire. Outside in the Orkney night the wind is dying too, and we are here together, alone in our island of tranquillity. Soon he will take off his glasses, put his feet on the sofa and fall asleep. He isn't sleeping well just now, always waking early, but he seems to have no problem dropping off.

'That pub we went to,' he said. 'It was like somebody's front room but with a bar all the way down one side. That's exactly what I expect Heaven to be like – if I get there.' He had found it during the day while I was working and, by his own account, spent some considerable time there. 'Do you remember the first time we were in Ireland?'

'When I was at that conference in Cork and it rained all the time?' It was more than twenty years ago that we were there together.

'And Anthony Clare was sitting at the next table at breakfast,' John laughs, 'I recognised his voice!' We both listened to him on *In the Psychiatrist's Chair* on the radio, quizzing celebrities about their lives. Rather different from the working life of most of my profession, but his fascinating explorations of their motivations was a reminder of why I had wanted to do the job. Listening to my patients, trying to understand and to help them.

'Life seemed simpler, then.'

'It was,' I reply, 'before things got difficult for both of us at work ... before you got so involved in caring for your parents.' I didn't mean it to come out quite that way.

He missed work at first, but he was the senior accountant and, when the company began to fail, they made him redundant. Like many men, his ability to earn defined him, but I hadn't realised quite how low he was until we watched a *Panorama* programme together about how middle-aged men can suddenly, and inexplicably, take their own lives. 'I know just how they felt,' he told me at the time.

He refused to see the doctor. Instead he drove up here to

spend some time alone, and a few days later I flew up to join him. We were so relieved to see each other in the terminal at Kirkwall airport we hugged and couldn't let each other go.

Losing your job, your income, sometimes your marriage, and even more so your self-respect. Keeping it all inside. Being a man. Just like my father had suffered in angry silence when things at home began to crumble. Going to bed for long periods after arguments with my mother. How irritable and down he was, but he never sought help. He carried on until he died, long before retirement age. He had no love for his job but continued as being in work was essential not just for the money but for his sense of self-worth. For many, the loss of the routine of work, being with other people and bringing home a wage even if your job is tedious, can even be fatal. John started to talk before his mood got too low but struggles to manage a different kind of working life now.

I switch off the TV, open a book, and leave him to nod off in front of the flickering embers, until he wakes up an hour later and goes to bed.

A few days later there is a disturbing newspaper article about the suicides of people who have had their benefits cut for failing to turn up at the job centre because they have been detained in hospital under the Mental Health Act or been undergoing cardiac surgery. People are starving to death or taking their own lives because of such a harsh approach to welfare.

Kyle was someone who I saw in his GP's surgery not so long before I retired, when this harsh regime began to bite. He arrived an hour late, looking very dishevelled and exhausted.

'I missed an appointment about my benefits the other

morning, because I can't get out of bed . . . I'm worried. They were stopped because they said I was fit for work, but I don't feel it.' He looked down at his hands and I could see that his nails were bitten down and ragged. 'There's no credit on my phone, and I've run out of my medication too . . . and I've got nothing to feed the dog with either.' He tried to smile but was on the verge of tears. 'What a state to get into, eh?'

'When did the community team last see you?'

'Oh, they discharged me a few months ago. I was managing OK for a while after that . . . ,' he paused for a moment as though distracted, 'Then the voices came back really loud, telling me what to do again like before . . . and not to listen to anyone.' He turned around looked up to the corner of the room for a moment, as though he was listening for some-thing I couldn't hear, then turned back to me, and carried on quickly, 'Can you do a letter for me for the benefits . . . I can't work, I can barely think . . . , they are telling me I shouldn't be speaking to you . . . please can you help me?'

There was much to do. Trying to get him back in touch with the mental health team: the voices had ordered him not to go when his GP had referred him again. Then completing more endless forms required by the Department of Work and Pensions to appeal against their decision on his benefit payments – whilst trying to support him in the meantime.

There are people in positions of power who seem to believe that being employed is the only therapy required for mental ill-health. We are back in the days of the deserving and undeserving poor, and those with severe mental illness, like Kyle, seem to fall into the latter group. He might not be in paid work, but that doesn't mean he is a person without worth.

These days, when not training others to do what I once did, I sit at my desk and write. No longer consulting, I am still contributing. Writing, arguing, campaigning for better mental health care. Not having to graft until the end as my parents did, I can create a new kind of 'work' on my own terms. Helping people who have mental health problems also aids my recovery without the conflicts and struggles of a regular job. Any job isn't better for your health than no job – in fact it can be worse. Getting back into that daily routine can be hard. It may take a while to reach the place which is right for you, and you can step off the treadmill and say, without having to apologise: 'I'm not feeling well. I simply cannot cope with work at the moment, but think I can begin to recover, if you give me time and the right kind of help.'

Looking up from my desk, at the view of Hoy, listening to John busying himself in the next room, I understand that I cannot go back.

John is driving me into Kirkwall this morning along the main road which follows the coast. The sea is choppy, and the tide is coming in fast, covering the rocky shore. In the distance a small ferry is emerging from the mist on its way back to Kirkwall from one of the other small islands, Rousay or Westray. In the summer you hold your breath to see if there is a cruise liner in port, rising from the sea like an incongruous floating block of flats, but they don't call at this time of year, in the dark days of January. There is a house on a tiny island along here that always fascinates me. It can only be reached by car at low tide along a track which curiously has a gate across it. At high tide the top of the gate above the water level is the only clue there is even a road there. I wonder what it is like to be completely cut off – probably one step too far for me.

'There must be otters living along this coast.' In so many ways it seems perfect for them, but I'm sad to say I've never seen an otter yet in Scotland. Wherever we travel I watch the shoreline in hope. Once, when we were on holiday, staying in a hotel room on Vancouver Island, next to the Pacific Ocean, John woke me from an afternoon nap. I often used to sleep away our holidays from work.

'Look, down there on the rocks.' He pointed to an otter and her two cubs returning from the ocean.

'Why don't we ever see them here?'

'Too many people nearby,' John suggests, 'And you need to get up earlier.'

'But there's a sign in Kirkwall near Tesco which says, "Otters crossing next 600 yards".' The supermarket is just across the road from a lake called the Peedie Sea, cut off from the big sea (peedie means 'small') by what was once a sandbank - the 'Ayre'. Before the town got busier it must have been a haven for otters.

'I expect they shop outside normal hours.'

'So, what are you going to do today?'

'Spend some time in the cathedral, then maybe go out to Scapa beach for a walk.' The light is not ideal for photography but I know how much he loves being able to wander, and the cathedral, with its warm, red sandstone walls that have stood for a thousand years always seems to beckon you inside for silent reflection, even if you are not a believer.

My meeting with one of the people involved in managing mental health services begins over a cup of tea. I open my notebook and ask what problems Orkney has with its mental health provision.

'So,' comes the reply, 'everyone agrees what we really need is a permanent consultant psychiatrist.'

There is a part of me that would love to be able to say, 'That's something I can do,' because that's true. I did it for more than thirty years until John told me, 'You cannot carry on any longer at this pace,' and he was right. It was never my patients who exhausted me – they are the ones I both miss and probably helped the most. The problem was having to deal with the bureaucrats and managers in the system.

I remember the pile of shredded paper and how I had disposed of the evidence that would be required to regain my licence to practise as a doctor. The temptation was foreseen.

'Well, I'm retired now but perhaps there is some other way I can help?'

CHAPTER 4

Escape

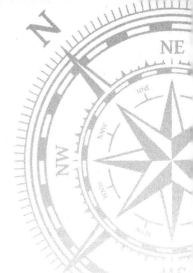

Early January brings a flurry of snow, but the Hoy hilltops are merely iced, not blanketed in white. From my desk window I can see green daffodil shoots poking through accumulations of snow on the lawn, and early buds appearing on the naked branches of the tree. A flock of graylag geese has settled on the field over the road, with more joining them by the minute. John has gathered his photography equipment by the front door, keen to get to the Ring of Brodgar before the snow begins to melt.

'Be careful,' I warn, 'The road might not have been gritted over there.'

'Don't worry!' He laughs, but I do. I cannot help myself.

Some problems over the last couple of months have been particularly troubling me. I agreed to go on television and talk about antidepressants, putting myself into the public world again when I didn't need to. Now I regret it, because of how I felt afterwards. I'd been on radio, but never TV. Live morning television, on a topic that everyone has an opinion on. It started with an email and a researcher from the BBC who said, 'It sounds like you might be a good person to have on the programme.'

What I had told her was that, not so long before, I asked my psychiatrist how I would have been over the last twenty years if I hadn't stayed on antidepressants. He thought I would have had at least one period of in-patient care. When I asked John, who remembers life before and after medication. His response was simple: 'You would be dead.'

For some people, antidepressants are helpful in improving mood. Others believe they are drugs of addiction and some see them as a way of 'numbing and sedating' emotional pain – a pharmacological means of escape.

Taking medication isn't an 'easy option'. It isn't just a medical decision; it can also be a moral one. On the one hand there is a doctor telling you to accept that you have an 'illness' and that if you take the required treatment you will be 'better' and able to carry on. On the other, you wonder 'is this really the right thing to do?' In explaining how depression is an 'illness', a professional tries to give you more hope and diminish your feelings of responsibility and guilt. Others see it as a way for doctors to impose a singularly medical view of what depression is. It's a difficult decision, deciding whether to take the tablets, when some are telling you not to.

Arriving early at Media City in Manchester, I sat with a cup of coffee, telling myself I didn't have to do this. Eventually, after going through security and being escorted to the relevant floor, I was fitted with a microphone. Perched on a chair with a projection of Salford Quays behind me, I could have been giving the weather forecast. Speaking into a camera, an image of me appeared on a wall of TV screens with other contributors in the studio in London. There were two other people 'on the wall' and a person being interviewed in the studio.

'Are you okay there?' asked the assistant in the studio, they will be coming to you soon.' A film was being shown about the serious problems that people had experienced both from taking antidepressants and trying to come off them. I had an opportunity to say a few words afterwards.

'On the occasions when I've taken antidepressants, they've helped me a great deal and taken me to a point where I could contribute again. I don't think I would be here now if I hadn't been able to take them.' This is what many people who have benefited from them think.

Antidepressants have helped me and others, but I prefer if people are given an informed choice. My patients expected me to have an opinion, but the final decision was theirs.

Several people pointed out afterwards on social media, and in a complaint to the BBC, that my viewpoint may be a biased one. During my career I have worked with 'big pharma',[6] even if I have, in order to stay well, taken the drugs of almost all the companies I collaborated with. How much has my contact with the drug industry influenced my views? I really don't know. Profit is the number one aim of the pharmaceutical industry, but antidepressants worked for me and for many of the patients I treated. Most psychiatrists (though not all) agree they are more effective than placebo pills. However, many are not helped, and some feel much worse when they are taking them.

I was on television for a minute at most. John called me to say he had watched it with his mother, and thought it went well.

'You got your point across, you were clear ... and passionate.'

The repercussions lasted much longer. I had not spoken so openly before about medication, and the criticisms levelled at me, my opinions, and the decision to invite me to speak on the programme, triggered my ruminative chorus of shame. *Am I really biased? What will people think of me? Why on earth did I do it?* Afterwards I just wanted to escape.

Driven to push myself into the glare, I often cannot cope with the, sometimes inevitable, consequences. I carry on wanting to speak about important things but am never prepared for the criticism that follows. Both my husband and my doctor ask me why I still do it.

In psychology 'an escape behaviour' is something you do to avoid a catastrophe that you fear is going to happen. I've never been comfortable telling someone they are doing the wrong thing by distracting themselves from anxious thoughts, but such actions can mean they never learn other ways to deal with it when some kinds of distraction can be life-saving: listening to music; watching television or a favourite DVD, so you don't have to think about the difficult meeting coming up next day. These ways of coping may not meet the gold standard of perfect psychological health but how much does that matter? We may not have faced up to all our problems, but sometimes we just have to find what works for us. Nevertheless, some ways of escape can be harmful.

In my younger days I escaped with alcohol but I'm more aware of the risks now. Alcohol is the unreliable friend of many who struggle with mood. We drink to console ourselves when we are sad and enhance the moment when we are happy. I am one of those who, as a GP colleague of mine once explained, are permanently short of two units of alcohol. I'm better company when I'm slightly under the influence, more sociable and relaxed.

Many people who are depressed start to drink at night to help them sleep. A Yorkshire housewife, previously teetotal, told me her neighbour across the garden fence had instructed her to, 'Have a whisky a night, its more natural than taking those sleeping pills.' A Scotsman would probably agree, but distilling is still a chemical process.

The trouble is that alcohol doesn't only take the edge off anxiety but opens a gateway to another level of consciousness where the hurt that other people inflict no longer seems important. However, not only does the despair return as the alcohol departs, but so does the physical pain the next day. I've met far too many people for whom alcohol dissolved their inhibitions about taking their lives, or some for whom intoxication with drugs was the ultimate escape from reality. One of my teachers described opiates, particularly heroin, as providing 'philosophical analgesia' and I thought how marvellous it would be to experience that, of course without getting hooked.

Barely surviving in a hovel, in a back street of a Northern town, a young couple declared to me once, 'There's nothing wrong with our lives,' as they huddled together in the darkness. 'We like living this way.' Their home looked like a set for an adaptation of Victorian novel. A bare mattress on the floor, an open fire with only cold ashes in the grate, even though it was an arctic day outside, and drug paraphernalia just visible under a filthy sheet. Difficult things had happened that they wanted to forget, but their mode of escape had resulted in a lifestyle only tolerable whilst out of their heads on heroin – which made a peculiar kind of sense.

This time I escaped, it did involve quite a lot of alcohol, but in the context of travelling, my other great way of fleeing life. A couple of weeks after the TV programme, I sat in an upgraded seat, bound for Rio de Janeiro, drinking champagne at 10 o'clock in the morning. I was getting away, escaping to a different world. On my way to a conference and to stay with a friend, I wasn't going to resist temptation. Time spent on a long-haul flight is like time off from the world. Suspended in the air, your life is on pause.

My Brazilian friend Sandra met me at the airport and drove us into the city along a road that has a sprawling favela on each side. The Olympics had finished a few weeks before, but the decorations and posters were still everywhere.

The opposite of depression isn't happiness but vitality: engaging with life, living life to the full, not dragging yourself along in the half-light of despair, and there are few people in the world with more vitality than Brazilians. I've learned, from previous visits, they are probably the noisiest people in the world. Once, shut in a hotel bathroom in Salvador, I struggled to hear John's voice on the telephone.

'They are practising for Carnival,' Sandra had shouted in my ear to explain, 'The real thing is even louder.'

I have known Sandra for more than twenty years now, and we have spent our lives doing similar kinds of work. That evening, she was remarkably phlegmatic about possibly not getting paid the next month because the local government in Rio, which funded the university, was broke. Despite all her problems she had bought a huge chocolate cake for my birthday, which we washed down with a bottle of warm pink

Brazilian champagne. In the hot airless night, I told her what had happened after the television appearance.

'Well, you know what drug companies are like,' she shrugged, 'They spend enough money on psychiatrists, do you remember that party you came to the first time you were in Brazil?'

Only too well. I had never been to one quite like it. Free booze and an unlimited buffet were paid for by pharmaceutical companies. It was the first and only time I saw a psychiatrist playing air guitar. It wasn't anything like the conference dinners I have been to at home. Do they spend that money to influence how doctors prescribe? Why would they do it, if it didn't work?

'That party ended up with an ambulance taking people away.'

I wasn't really listening. 'I worry that people think I am dishonest.'

'You worry too much, but then so do I . . . eat and drink, forget about it the Brazilian way!'

For a few hours it worked. Alcohol is a solvent that dissolves memories and pain. Until the next day.

I hear the door open and look up. It is almost lunchtime, and John has arrived back home, letting a cool breeze into the kitchen.

'It's wonderful up there, and I am going to get you away from this desk.'

'How busy is it?'

'Not like the summer, but everyone seems to be enjoying the snow.' His hands are freezing in the fingerless gloves I gave him for photography.

an I come tomorrow? I'm in the middle of something.'

ie thinks I spend far too long at my desk. It is easier to ite when he isn't here, but then I miss his company.

When I was very young, I would travel everywhere I could with Dad. We delivered the children's rides he helped design and build when he was in business with a friend. Shaped like animals and speedboats, you put sixpence in a slot and they rocked backwards and forwards for a couple of minutes. It was as if the two of us were escaping together.

Trips to Birmingham always remind me how we delivered those rides to the spanking new Bull Ring Shopping Centre in its 1960s heyday, before it became grungy, neglected, and condemned as Brutalist rather than 'modern'. A memento of that journey, the official guide to the Centre filled with the architect's drawings of figures travelling up and down huge escalators, was my childhood image of what city life would be like. Clean, well-organised and safe with lots of shops. Unlike the reality when I would be followed home by a stranger in the early hours, get threatened by drunks and have my car broken into.

We set off in the middle of one night for Bristol, sitting high in the cab of the Ford pick-up which smelled of plastic seat covers and dusty fibre-glass resin from the factory. Behind us, just visible through the rear window of the cab were shapes wrapped in sheets and tied with string. After delivering the rides in the morning we wandered about the city centre, rebuilt, like Birmingham, in wall-to-wall concrete after the second world war. Dad bought me an atlas which I kept for years until it fell apart, travelling in dreams inside that book. Later, we looked over the Clifton Gorge from the suspension bridge and ate ice cream at the zoo, enjoying our time out from the day-to-day grind of school and work.

My family rarely took holidays before I left home. Through most of my childhood we were marooned on the East coast of England but during a stay with family in Scotland, Dad said, 'Plan us a route to the Highlands that we can do in a couple of days.'

I cannot remember very much of that trip, which is odd because it was so important to me, the farthest away from home I had ever been. We stopped to eat in a café in the village of Kinlochleven where we were served a fry-up by a very dour waitress. As we came into Fort William, Mum pointed out all the 'vacancies' on Bed and Breakfast signs, which were everywhere in late September, but Dad kept driving until we reached Glen Nevis, where we all spent a freezing cold night in the car. I don't think I quite understood that my parents probably wanted to avoid the expense of lodgings because they had no money. No wonder they were stressed and unhappy.

When I was a teenager, we spent a week in a cabin near Loch Ness and collected fresh creamy milk each morning from the post-office in whisky bottles, which still held the faint scent of spirits. My younger brother Alan, seeing a stag's head mounted on the wall in the post office asked, 'Is it standing behind the wall? Has it just put its head through?' He had never seen a hunting trophy.

Before returning south, we visited Glen Affric, one of the most beautiful glens in Scotland, where Dad took photographs of the loch, capturing the forested slopes and clear blue sky for posterity. I wish I had that picture now. A couple of years ago, I went back to rediscover the glen, only to find it had been invaded by a horde of campervans which seemed to be breeding somewhere at the end of the road. I wanted to relive the tranquillity of that day in the 1960s but spent most of my time passing oncoming traffic, not so much escaping urban life as re-joining it. There isn't sufficient space to accommodate even a mini in a passing place on a single-track road in Glen Affric when a campervan is juddering towards you.

Over half a century has passed, and I am still travelling. Since I opened the atlas for that first time to explore the world with my fingertips, I have taken every opportunity my occupation gave me. Whenever I attended a conference or was invited to teach, I would take time to explore on my own. In every place, whether in a frozen Siberian city or the balmy warmth of Southern California, it has felt as if I have not only been trying to escape but searching for where I truly belong: my cabin with peace of mind, my place of escape and hibernation, where I don't have to live in the real world.

Whilst visiting Sandra in Rio, I struggled, as ever, with the heat and humidity covering myself in a sticky combination of tropical strength insect repellent and factor 30 sun block. By the time we arrived at the Samba bar for the evening our week's work was done. My superego was chased away by the first two Caipirinhas of the evening and my body responded to the music.

As a small child, I loved dancing. I must have been about five years old when l was jumping around in front of the radiogram, watched by my amused parents. Later, at a birthday party, another girl said, 'That's not dancing! That's just silly!'

I don't remember telling Mum and Dad, I don't know why, but instead I harboured a sneaking suspicion that was what they thought too. That painful self-awareness remains but has never stopped me on the dance floor. I overcame my anxiety about dancing when I discovered nobody else cares what I look like. I could escape into the rhythm and lose myself.

I remember a Saturday night in the 1970s at the Sheffield Polytechnic Union swirling around the dance floor to Steve Harley and Cockney Rebel in a full-length purple skirt. I was visiting my school friend, Heather, who was studying there. Having just broken up with my first serious boyfriend, I was determined to prove that it wasn't the end of the world, but I was so alone and despairing. Each morning I got out of bed in my room in the Pollock Halls of Residence in Edinburgh, and stared at the view of Arthur's Seat and the Salisbury Crags. A wonderful vista, but without a single human being in sight. I felt that if I disappeared from the world no one would miss me. At the end of an interminable spring term I escaped on the railway down to Sheffield and we went to the Saturday night disco. By the end of the evening I was sitting on the lap of a guy I had met on the dance floor.

Heather exclaimed, 'I don't think I've ever seen you like this before!'

Here was the class swot, the good girl, who was so happy to be alive after such an acute sense of loss and beckoning loneliness, but who in her heart knew she had only temporarily dissolved it in alcohol.

As we grow older and time passes, the illusion of carefree youth intensifies. In those early months of 1975, my new life in Edinburgh was far from stable as I struggled to deal with mixed feelings about leaving home: anxiety and yet relief from escaping a family – and particularly a father – from whom I felt increasingly alienated. Those few hours on a dance floor, lost in the beat, offered some relief from the world before I had to go on trying to be an adult.

So, in the crush of the dance floor in Rio, the familiar rhythms of the city pulsed again. For these two hours, not having to ruminate about what I should or should not have said or done, I was possessed by the music and unable to stop moving until I was so exhausted, I had to sit down.

'Are you okay?' Sandra asked. She had been dancing with a man on the other side of the floor.

'You two looked very good together!' I told her.

'Yeah, but he's an Argentinian . . . They think they are so much better than us . . . but they aren't!' She looked at me and sighed. My clothes were soaked with perspiration.

'I just want a long glass of water and my bed,' I laughed, 'Let's go home.'

'You may be English, but you have the soul of a Brazilian,' someone said to me once on a dance floor in Brazil. I so wished he had been right.

One of the common ways we run away from ourselves is by running into relationships. So many of my patients over the years have done this, particularly women. By investing in a relationship, often with a partner as wounded as themselves, sometimes more so and capable of inflicting real harm, many people try to heal by pouring energy and love into another person. In this dangerous kind of love, too often the loved one is not as they appeared through the rose-tinted lenses of need and desire, and emotional, physical and even sexual abuse can result. Repeating the events of traumatic child-hoods can confirm negative self-images in an ever-repeating cycle of despair.

From the moment I left home to go to University, I repeated this pattern. Trying to relieve the emptiness with the warm glow that comes from the attention of a person who seemed, at first, to want to be with me. He was older than me, experienced and funny. We were both studying medicine, but he had done a degree before. As so many others do when they are desperate for love, I pretended to be something I wasn't. Escaping into the persona of a more confident and mature person I professed to enjoy our lifestyle of heavy drinking and sex, an act that can only be maintained for so long. In fact, both of us were avoiding being our true selves. When he said he wanted to end the relationship because I 'wasn't fun to be with any more', I escaped into alcohol and the next liaison. There is a song from that time that plays to the memory of those grey mornings when I had to drag myself into university, echoing what I was telling myself, *I'm not in love*. Each time I found myself in the same place I simply tried harder.

Working in towns with universities, I saw several young women during my career who escaped in similar ways. Kelly, a first-year student, was accompanied to see me by her best friend who looked very concerned about her. However, Kelly's opinion was different. 'She's completely fed up with me, everyone is.'

'Why is that?' I asked.

'I'm just driving them all crazy. Since I broke up with my last boyfriend, they think I've gone mad,' she whispered through tears. 'I've been getting drunk all the time, bingeing on food . . . they don't know what to do with me any more. All they say is, "he was an idiot anyway so you're better off without him".'

Kelly had been harming herself too, cutting her skin repeatedly with a razor blade on her forearms, making short and determined gashes until she bled. Not only as a way of coping with the pain of being alive, but at times just to feel something, anything to fill the awful emptiness inside her. 'They've taken me up to the hospital a couple of times, but I've said I'll never go back there again, they were horrible to me.' Sadly, I wasn't surprised. People who harm themselves are sometimes treated as wasting medical and nursing time. Not only cruel, it disregards their much higher risk of suicide.

Before she had left home, Kelly had been in therapy with someone from the young peoples' mental health services. It helped, but unfortunately ended when she turned eighteen. What she needed was a decent therapist once more. Someone who would care if she lived or died.

That was what I benefited from, and with the help of both therapy and good fortune (and the cats who discovered that the man living two doors along was an easy mark), I was able to love, and be loved in return.

No two places could contrast more than Orkney in winter and the favela Sandra had worked in for several years, providing mental health care for the residents and much needed support for the family doctors. A favela is a shanty town, usually built on a hillside, where people live without the usual services of water, sewerage, and mains electricity. In Rio you can be in one of the smarter middle-class areas of town but only a stone's throw from the shanties on the hillsides.

I was not prepared for the sensual assault of the favela. Two healthcare workers escorted us as it wouldn't have been safe to go alone. The sun was frying my brain from above and the smell of dirt and human waste rose from beneath our feet. Wary eyes watched us over half built balconies as we made our way slowly past armed police officers lounging like mangy cats in the heat. Children played in the concrete park halfway up the hillside and one of our group covertly snapped a photograph of the electricity supply pole with all the illegal connections hanging precariously from it. We had been warned against taking pictures because of the risk of inadvertently including someone wanted by the police in the frame. Two feral cats slept by the edge of a foul stream of water. The shriek of a woman's voice pierced through the beat of rap music. There was an awful feeling of unease.

We emerged from the cabins back onto the streets and with a rush of relief inhaled the polluted but less fetid air. The health workers showed us their clinic. There were spaces on their noticeboard where they recorded chronic illnesses. No surprise to see words for TB, diabetes and hypertension, the most common problems there. Living in fear has a lasting impact on your blood pressure.

'You still try to make a difference,' I said to Sandra. Part of me envied her. For all my training, I felt somehow useless in comparison.

She knew the mother and daughter who had served lunch to us earlier in the local Samba school. 'Both of them are struggling – they've had difficult relationships, violence in the family, but I'm so pleased with how things are going for them now. They help at the school. It's where everyone practices for Carnival.'

That is the time when everyone in the favelas of Rio marches and dances through the street, and escapes for a few short days, from reality. With cruel irony, I was present as a tourist but also a voyeur, escaping the stresses of my privileged life, in a place where millions of people were trapped by accident of birth, race and fortune in appalling poverty.

Here in Orkney, like everywhere else in the world, life can be hard if you are poor, alone, or both. All over the world, small and isolated communities can be harsh places if you do not fit in.

Is it wrong to want to run away from your problems? Does running away help you recover, and from the awful low moods they trigger? Sometimes it is lifesaving. We don't all have the strength, courage and stamina to face our demons and deal with them. It can take time. If you have been ground down you may need some 'time out' to regain hope for the future, or simply protect yourself and those who matter to you. Many will not find the process of recovery straightforward. When you are poor, homeless or traumatised by past and present it can be simply too much to overcome.

We walk with care on snow which has fallen on the slippery tracks of the people who walked up this path to visit the stones yesterday. Parts of the track are roped off at this time of year, to give the turf a chance to recover from the battering it has taken during the summer months.

John is reminiscing. 'Last summer when I was up here, one minute I could see far and wide as the sun was setting. There were people everywhere, but soon after they left the mist swirled in. It was just me and the ancient stones.'

A chilly breeze disturbs the gunmetal grey surface of the

loch as we walk towards the great stones that have stood here for millennia, as long as Stonehenge, maybe even longer. Graceful swans and their cygnets, no longer ugly ducklings, glide as always near the shoreline. Off the path, frozen puddles are covered with thin ice and soak my feet when I kick my heels in, but I am fascinated by the random patterns that ice makes as it breaks sometimes into clean, straight lines, but at other times transformed by water and air trapped beneath into curious shapes.

'It isn't enough for you, is it?' John knows me too well. 'You want more from life.'

'I still want to be useful. To be needed.' That's it, or some of it. 'Maybe I don't just need to recover from depression, I have to recover from being a doctor.'

He chides me for dillydallying, 'Let's get back and get warm.'

In a couple of weeks, we will travel south again, John to his responsibilities. Cover has been arranged with a carer to go into his mother each day, and his sister has put in extra hours, as he does when she takes a break.

I have plenty to do but my mood still hasn't really recovered. Each time I've relapsed in the last few years, my medication has been changed. I'm on a combination of tablets again. Last time I saw my psychiatrist he raised the possibility of seeking more therapy, but I rejected that idea. I don't want to spend any more time digging over the past. However, escape only works for so long. Eventually you must face the problems you are running away from. We can spend too much of our lives avoiding who we are. I have found writing helpful, and now I want to explore other ways of becoming and staying as well as I can. Does the anguish of depression inspire great work or is mental illness the antithesis of creative achievement? For me, no kind of creativity is possible without medication but, when I am overmedicated, I struggle to find the energy to think. Life without pills cannot be managed.

When you run to escape the problems in your head, they tend to travel along with you. Trying to transform your island to match that fantasy of the perfect bolt hole doesn't work. Through the work I've been doing here I have discovered that Orkney, too, has its problems: one of the highest alcohol consumptions in Scotland, and a high rate of suicide, despite being regularly listed as one of the most desirable places in the United Kingdom. A fellow psychiatrist told me how he spends twice as much time per head of population caring for folks with problems who live on one of the inner Hebridean Islands than those who reside in a town on the mainland. Many of the islanders are incomers for whom the realities of island life don't meet their expectations. A former colleague told me how much his friend loved living in Skye but was leaving to return to Glasgow, because she couldn't tolerate the wind any more, it was driving her crazy. The Northern Isles would most definitely not be the place for her.

Leaving now, closing the car door, John tells me, 'I always miss being here. It feels such a long way from everything going on at home.'

The light is fading in the west and Orkney will soon be in darkness again.

CHAPTER 5

Being kinder to myself

Spring is on its way but hasn't yet arrived in Orkney. It is cold and wet with a mist rising over the land which has been swirling in from the sea since yesterday, muffling the Wee Hoose from the outside world. The daffodils in my garden are still in bud, while down in the south they will be well into flower.

'You are still sitting at that desk too much,' John said on the phone this morning.

He's been telling me that, repeatedly. I always agree with him, but don't change my ways. He would be annoyed if I told him I have been finishing off some academic work rather than continuing with my own writing. Not wanting to desert them, I'm still in touch with a couple of my doctoral students from the university who haven't yet submitted their theses.

This time I let his words pass without comment. 'What do you think about getting someone to look at the front windows? I think they've had it.' Household matters are easier.

Living where the changing seasons are so visible in the landscape helps to anchor me in the real world. The longer evenings are full of promise as the earth comes back to life. Fields are gradually changing from the umber and blackish browns of winter to shades of olive and even emerald green, especially when April showers have been heavy. Everywhere there are deep pools of rainwater that may delay the date when the cows can graze outside again.

You barely notice seasons in the city. In Manchester the weather was simply wet, dry, warm or cold in any combination. Yet I do remember taking the train back to the suburbs, just after my birthday in November, and watching the autumn smog coalesce around particles of smoke rising from the Guy Fawkes bonfires. Not having a garden, I was never consciously aware of the arrival of spring and too preoccupied to notice the buds on the few neighbourhood trees. In our garden in Yorkshire, the flowering cherry will bloom for only a few sweet days before shedding her clusters of tiny pink bouquets across the garden path. Those delicate petals wouldn't survive for more than a few seconds in the Orkney wind. Flora and fauna must be hardier to thrive here. It's not a forgiving climate.

Like the changing seasons, recovery can be delayed and unpredictable. Getting the right treatment is only the beginning. Then you have to think about how to stop it happening again and minimise its impact if it returns. You may believe it is an 'illness', perhaps some kind of 'disability', with treatment that you simply have to 'survive' and which you may not have wanted anyway. I can identify with each of these points of view, although I've never been forced to have medication or go into hospital.

All I do know is that I don't feel strong at the moment and certainly not resilient. Not 'recovered', yet I'm still pushing myself too hard. Why? All my life I have been striving to succeed. I was the oldest child in my family, and I started at a small private school at the age of three. Later I found out that my mother resented the expense. 'The council school was good enough for my kids,' our GP told her on one of her many visits. By the time I was five I was reading well and taking piano lessons. Dad helped me memorise all those facts you have to regurgitate in geography exams, and I can still draw a map of the coalfields of Britain. Getting 99 per cent in tests wasn't good enough for Dad, but Mum just didn't see the point. She would go to parents' evenings alone while Dad and I waited at home. He would make the excuse that it would take too long to clean himself up after work, but I think anxiety was his real reason. Sometimes it felt good to hear from Mum that my teachers thought I had talent and would get to university. At other times, it felt as though my success just embarrassed her.

'The headmaster says he's fed up of hearing your name from other parents,' she said, at the end of my first year at grammar school.

Mum's work colleague, Kath, saw things differently. Mum had been delighted when I learned how to make dresses at school. Kath let me use her old treadle sewing machine.

As she sat in the easy chair next to me as I sewed, sharing a packet of Marks and Spencer's jam tarts between us and her overweight Labrador, she said, 'We know someone who is in your class who lives down the road, and she goes on about how easy it is for you ... but I told her how hard you study ... don't you?'

She was right. Sometimes until the early hours.

The decision to take science subjects came after Mum

reported back, 'The English teacher said you worked very hard, but would never write anything original.' Medicine seemed the best to aim for. By getting a job at the end of my degree I could escape home and gain my independence. Dad didn't make it to my graduation either. At the party afterwards, my mother-in-law brought up the discussion of where my then husband, who was finishing a PhD, might work. He mentioned the Atomic Energy Authority. 'Do you mean Dounreay?' she asked, 'That would be a good place wouldn't it?'

Dounreay was Scotland's first nuclear reactor, on the north coast and not so far from here. Now it is being demolished, piece by piece, but it had great cachet before we learned that it had been polluting the ocean for years with nuclear waste. The same ocean that washes Orkney's beaches.

'But I wouldn't be able to get a job there . . . ' I butted in.

'Your husband's going to be the breadwinner now!' my mother-in-law replied, and my mother, standing alongside her, nodded.

It seemed that I had a problem of over-ambition. Much later, I realised Carl Jung was right about 'wounded healers'. In caring for others, we try to deal with the damaged, unresolved issues of our early lives. We don't consider how the simple act of 'helping people' might be hazardous to both our physical and mental health when practised with perfectionist fervour. Being a doctor licensed me to take care of others while trying (and eventually failing) to suppress my own needs for love and care, which had only been partially met by my father and, more or less, failed by my mother.

Spring is here but the cows are still in their barns, bellowing across the valley. They spend all winter indoors where my neighbour has to constantly provide silage to feed them. I hear his tractor each time it trundles to the barn up the lane behind my house. There are no other sounds except for the tapping of the rain on the skylight above my head, the breeze gusting across the chimney pots amplified by the open door of the cold stove in the hearth. Following instructions from a meditation course, I focus attention on my breath as it flows into my lungs and out again, catching slightly at the back of my throat. I am beginning to feel connections again, between my body and my 'self' and then between my 'self' and the world; the first time I have experienced that sense of peace for some weeks.

The current answer to everything from stress at work to full blown depression and even psychosis seems to be Mindfulness. At a lecture in Manchester, a couple of years ago, given by one of the people who came up with the idea, I learned how combining mindfulness with cognitive therapy isn't a treatment for acute depression, but it can prevent relapse. My own therapist taught me some of these skills: how to allow problematic thoughts to move in and out of immediate consciousness. So, despite my initial scepticism, I have been finding it helpful to listen to a guided meditation on *self-compassion – being kind to yourself*. When the narrator asks me to focus on my pain and allow myself to experience it, a great well of sadness opens inside me and the tears flow. As when I've had an argument with someone who is important to me, crying brings relief as I recognise those feelings and where they originate. However, it only works when I am stable and calm to begin with.

After writing a blog recently about my views on

mindfulness, I heard from many people about their experiences, both good and bad. One person told me, 'I'd been chronically depressed for years, and mindfulness has really helped me tremendously.' Another: 'It really has changed my life! I used to worry about what was going to happen all the time. I don't do that now I just focus on the present.' However, a former colleague contacted me to say, 'When I was really anxious and depressed, a psychologist tried to get me to do it. It just didn't have any impact at all on how I was feeling, even though he was enthusiastic about it. He just kept telling me, "This is something that's going to put the pharmaceutical companies out of business".' Hearing that, I did wonder how much time he had spent with people who were in severe distress. Another said, 'When my community nurse mentions it these days, I just growl.' When very low, focusing on your anxiety, worries and ruminations can make you feel even worse.

Some also objected to the way that Mindfulness is promoted for personal self-fulfilment far removed from Buddhism's intention of compassion. Or as a corporate tool to help employees work more efficiently: with greater 'resilience'. Neither of these ends is in harmony with the ethics and morals of Buddhist belief. 'For those of us who encountered the idea of mindfulness through our involvement with Buddhism,' a person wrote, 'it's as if we are talking two different languages'. He explained how he wouldn't dream of recommending it to anyone – people have to recognise and accept, for themselves, their innate ability to be present in the moment. Putting this learning into practice, I have begun to manage my own thinking a little more effectively.

Since retiring, I still go to London occasionally to spend

a day teaching doctors about suicide prevention. Last year, I was preoccupied with my own relentlessly negative thoughts before travelling down: *Why are you still doing this? No-one wants to hear what you have to say. You don't work on the front line any more; you don't even work at all. They won't take you seriously . . . they will just laugh at you. You are a fake.*

The railway journey from Sheffield to London was slow, stopping almost everywhere. In Nottingham the ageing diesel train entered the station in one direction and reversed out again. My forward-facing seat became 'away' from the direction of travel: *that's fine – can I just go back again?* When I reached the modern hotel in the East End, I couldn't get a mobile signal in my room. Standing outside with the smokers in a freezing cold wind, the only place the network seemed to function, I telephoned John. 'I'm fine. Really.' I lied. 'Just very tired.'

I have always felt like an imposter who is about to be found out. I don't have to carry on doing this, but in a strange way, it serves rather like a treatment programme for a phobia. If I completely avoided exposure I would never set foot in an academic department or on stage at a conference. So, I continue to *feel the fear and do it anyway*, knowing that each event inoculates me against panic and subsequent avoidance. One way to recover from depression is to simply keep going. Not to retreat from life. If I act better, it does help me to feel better too.

Next morning, I was tense and edgy, aware of the body language and comments of one or two members who thought they had nothing else to learn.

'What's new about this? It's really for beginners isn't it?'

is everyone always wanting to talk about communi-
...ion. I know how to talk to patients!'

I never had that confidence in my ability, particularly
with someone who was unsure about trusting me and
fearful that they might be detained against their will in
hospital. When you are deeply depressed your thinking
possesses a warped logic of its own. You see the world in
half-light with long shadows, a place that might be better
off without you, where your exit from a dark corner might
even go unnoticed. Where you want to be both dead and
alive at the same time.

The day passed quickly and, absorbed in listening, talking
and explaining to others, I became distracted from my fears
and worries. Through acting like a competent person my
mood lifted and I coped, even with disagreements.

I was told by one doctor. 'Our psychologist says we should
tell people to practice what they've learned about mindfulness when they are in a crisis.'

'Well it worries me,' I shrugged, 'Because people tell us it
really doesn't help.' I went on, 'It's often coupled with advice
such as: Have a nice cup of tea, or a warm bath, or take your
dog for a walk.' I recalled someone on the blog saying what
she wanted at such difficult times wasn't to feel patronised.
Just for someone to, 'Simply be there, listen, accept and not
judge me.'

On the train home I resisted the ruminative thoughts that
always plague me after a day spent with other people. Some
people imagine potential worries floating past in little boxes,
and let them go past, but that doesn't work for me. Each
one is a tempting Pandora's box and sometimes, when I
cannot find a reason for my anxiety, I reach for one as it flies

past. What then though? I stack them on the top shelf of my mental closet, out of the way.

The other week, a nurse told me how she had been instructed by a manager not to 'get too close to your patients. It encourages dependence.' She was worried that one particular patient was being discharged too soon, as many people are.

I've been fortunate so far, but a few weeks ago I received a letter from the hospital where I currently visit my psychiatrist. The words jumped out from the page . . . *Our plans to stop some of our services* . . . It wasn't entirely a surprise. It's a specialist service for people with complex mood disorders. The man I see there knows more about medication for mood problems than anyone I have seen before and has supported me through the last couple of years. I'm worried that he may have to stop seeing me.

As a doctor, I tried to bend the system to fit the person rather than insist on compliance with the status quo. I remember a female colleague saying, 'I'm not prepared to see women who want to see a woman doctor; if her consultant is male, well that's not my problem.' I didn't share her opinion. Given what we know now about how many women with mental health problems have experienced sexual abuse I am not surprised that so many wanted to talk to a female. I've seen men who would only talk to a woman for the same reason. I tried to provide what people needed, when they needed it, knowing it is hard to say to your employer, 'I need time to go and see a doctor regularly for my mind.'

The idea that 'kindness is a virtue of losers' is a relatively modern phenomenon. Being capable of bearing the vulnerability of other people, and therefore facing up to our own frailties, is something people are ambivalent about.

Years ago, when I worked in a mental health ward, other staff were at first very sympathetic towards a patient of mine, Claire, who was very depressed. She had been abused by her stepfather, and more recently beaten by her boyfriend. After the suicide of a close friend she tried to take her own life.

Showing sympathy to someone involves merely imagining what your life would be like in similar circumstances. You are so relieved that you demonstrate your sympathy with kindness and attention.

When Claire's oldest daughter came to visit it was clear that she missed her mother very much. Claire cried because she couldn't be with her family. Still feeling sympathetic, the staff comforted her, as much as they could. When Claire was told that her younger children were being taken into care she reacted, violently and unexpectedly, by cutting herself. 'I'm useless,' she said. 'I shouldn't be here.'

'Why did you cut yourself? Why didn't you ask for help?' a nurse asked.

'Because you don't care. You only pretend. No-one does really.'

Claire became angrier and that evening tried to hang herself. No-one had ever, in her experience, really cared for her though many had pretended to. When a member of staff questioned her motives, rather harshly, by asking, 'Did you do it for attention? Because you weren't talking to us yesterday,' she became even more alienated and the fragile connection was broken.

At this point the ward staff became markedly less sympathetic and their kindness evaporated. Claire was no longer behaving like a 'good' patient, grateful for their help and care.

No-one wanted to sit down with her and ask, 'What does it feel like?' To show empathy, you have to understand how a person sees themselves, their world and their future within it, even if you disagree with how they are behaving. Being kind to someone who is struggling with their own internal turmoil, risks putting you in touch with your own unhappiness and suffering. It wasn't long before someone mentioned the words 'personality disorder'. If my own therapists had not tried so hard to understand me, I could have easily been given that diagnosis too.

Yet, sitting with Claire I found her wanting to talk as long as others wanted to hear, without judging her. How can you learn to treat yourself with kindness and compassion if you have no idea what that means? As a young doctor, assuaging my thirst to be needed, I found it all too easy to understand my patients' difficulties because I was already confused and there was little difference between us.

Providing the compassion and understanding they needed came at considerable cost to me. Exhausted, I still didn't feel 'good enough' and pushed myself even harder.

'What have you been doing today?' John asks. It's Skype time and I am missing him even though I know that if he was with me, he would disapprove of how much I'm working.

'Oh, just getting this book finished off.'

'Which one?'

'The textbook.' It's a second edition. A copy of the first, co-written with colleagues, one of whom sadly died not long after its publication, sits prominently on the bookshelf next to me. 'If I ever agree to do a third edition of this will you please take that as evidence that I've finally lost it.'

'You haven't been getting much of your own writing done then?'

I can hear his disapproval and change the subject. 'Any news on your mother?'

'Yes. We went to visit the home yesterday.'

'How did it go? Did she like it?' It is a silly question.

In the last month, my mother-in-law has finally accepted that she needs to go into care. She wanted John and his sister to keep on providing ever more intensive care for her in her own home, but this could not go on. I can see the impact it is having on John. 'You look tired, what time did you get back?' I ask.

'Late afternoon. I couldn't get away. I used to feel so guilty, but now I'm starting to get angry and I hate that.' He is finding it hard to be kind to himself too. 'I'm looking forward to you coming back to Yorkshire again,' he says. There is a wistfulness in his voice that threatens to lever up the lid on the well of tears that I try to keep firmly in place. 'Take some time off the work and get out for the day.'

What he means is get some exercise. I know he is right but can't admit it. My mood is so up and down at the moment. I should be happier that John has kept his promise about the two years that he made to me. Now we can make our own plans, but part of me still feels as though my heels are dug into the ground while the rest of me tries to move forwards.

Over the last few days, when it hasn't been pouring with rain, I have driven several times to our nearest beach, Waukmill Bay, a quiet place known only to dog walkers and other wandering locals. Last summer, we came across a nimble red-brown stoat on this road carrying something which looked like a mouse in his mouth. Standing his ground in front of the car for a moment he turned a couple of summersaults and disappeared into the nearest field.

'That was amazing, was he showing off?' John had braked to avoid him.

Stoats aren't native to the islands and prey on ground-nesting birds, and the Orkney Vole, which is a unique sub-species, was possibly what our roadside performer had just caught. No-one knows how they got here but they've only been seen in the last few years.

I wonder if they attack young cats? At least there are no foxes in Orkney. Like me he is another interloper here, but one that is unwelcome.

Close by a strand of cottages, it is the only place nearby where the shore can be reached at high tide. A long descent through abundant yellow gorse leads to a shallow bay by the stream from the old mill. On the opposite side the slope is steep and rocky, and when the tide comes in the sands are covered and a network of shifting sandbars reminds me of the beaches where I grew up in England. Another path cuts down the grey rock face nearer the sea but can only be used when the tide is out, and I haven't found an easy way across the marshland between the beach and the main road.

Clambering down broad steps edged with old logs, slippery and wet from the recent rain, eventually onto the sand, is exhilarating. The mist has cleared, but the clouds are thickening, and the temperature could be a few degrees warmer despite a short visit from the sun an hour ago. This evening, as the fog drifts in, it is a curiously eerie experience to be completely folded into the cloud, a grey walled space containing only me, pale yellow sand and water, with no sound but the waves lapping on the shore.

I don't linger on the beach. I don't think I have ever felt so completely alone, and it reminded me of the feeling of being trapped inside my head during my last serious relapse. Climbing over the brow of the hillside to the road, I am relieved by signs of real, ongoing life, even if one of the older houses is gradually being reclaimed by nature. This is the world that I want to be part of.

Unable to write much of late, I have been reading. With so much more available time I can concentrate when alone, but I have been trying to understand why I still struggle with my emotions. Insights from therapy are still arriving years later and, as I read, ideas begin to form. Some are easily dismissed but others help to make sense of the world. Reading as therapy is called *Bibliotherapy* and there are plenty of books out there to go on, although now that British bookshops have adopted the American term *mind, body and spirit* the selection can be somewhat eclectic, ranging from assertiveness training to crystal therapy. All are described in detail in the old paperback sitting on my bookshelf, with the grandiose title *The Encyclopedia of Reality*. A book is cheaper than therapy, and easier to obtain. It provides not only information, but also hope, inspiration and things to be done that can solve your problems and move you towards your own idea of recovery.

Reading about how people who have experienced a harsh and shaming upbringing can find it difficult to care about themselves helps me to understand myself a little more. I'm still trying to regain the affection of my father and recover from my mother's anger and disappointment.

However, some writers will tell you that there is a single,

simple answer to your problem and that worries me. Inferring that what has happened to you is essentially your own fault, that you must be weak and unmotivated, they appeal most to those who believe in being cruel to be kind. Many of the things that cause us difficulty in life are not under our control. Self-help books can be useful but if you are severely depressed it can be hard to motivate yourself to open them, which is one of the reasons I find the title of one of them, *The Way Out of Your Prison*, so problematic. It clearly works for some, as sometimes we have to be pushed to make changes in our lives, but for me, knowing that the person cajoling me to change really cares, and that I can trust them, is what matters.

What has enabled me to learn what it means to be kinder to myself has been the compassionate friendship, love and care of others.

This week there was an e-mail from my friend in Seattle, who I'm looking forward to seeing later in the year. I used to believe that it would be difficult to make new friendships later in life, but in the years since I completed therapy I've made some that are very close.

Eighteen years ago, I went to live and work in America for a year. When John told our neighbour in South Yorkshire that I was going away, she asked, 'Are you going to let her?'

'I don't think I can stop her,' he said. 'Anyway, why would I want to?'

'If my husband said that I would tell him not to bother coming back . . . '

She didn't understand our relationship. Her expectations of married life were quite different.

Reflecting on the experience, it feels almost like a practice run, a taster of how life might be when I had time to recover completely from depression. My friend Loryn contributed a great deal to that. She was my landlady in the bohemian city of Seattle in the far North West of the United States, with a climate rather like Manchester, but much better scenery. Mount Rainier was visible most days as the trolley bus descended past the Space Needle to the city centre. From my office on the eighteenth floor of a tower block downtown, the mountains of the Olympic Peninsula beckoned across the sparkling water of Puget Sound.

On first arrival, as the yellow cab drove North along the waterfront highway, the Alaskan Way, against the spectacular backdrop of the city lights to the East and Pacific to the West, I wondered how on earth I would fit into this alien place. At the bottom of steps to a painted wooden house which looked like it had blown in from Scandinavia I met Loryn, a university administrator who had decided to let out the basement of her family home. Since I had no clue about social security cards, transport, where to shop, how to have fun, she took me under her wing.

'Would you like to go for a walk into town?' she came downstairs to ask me a few days later. 'How are you managing down here, are you OK?'

'I'd ... love to!' I said, with a little uncertainty. 'I'm fine really.'

The apartment was compact but warm and comfortable, with a desk and lamp in the corner of the living room, a place where I could concentrate on writing, which I had been unable to do before arriving. What I hadn't prepared for was for someone interested in me as a person. She wanted to get to know me and, soon, I her. That was the beginning of an exploration of the city and, over the years, many other places.

When John came to visit at Christmas, he couldn't believe how well I looked. We hugged at the arrival gate. 'You look ten years younger!' he cried. In the innocent months before 9/11 you could still meet a person directly off the plane.

I tried to keep up those interests for several years, but then work took over again. Loryn chided me for not keeping in touch, and I realised that she not only cared about me but wanted to build a long-lasting friendship. She feels like the older sister I never had. Her gift, a tiny red shoe with a delicate stiletto heel, is on the shelf above my laptop screen. We both so love shoe shopping.

'I couldn't believe how different you were when I came to see you that time in Seattle,' John says every now and then.

The problem is that sometimes I cannot believe it either, so much has happened since then. I need to give myself permission to become that person again.

Our society is so ambivalent about kindness. We are constantly told how we should take greater responsibility for ourselves, however unwell we happen to be, rather than be dependent on the state. Our society that has become ever harsher, with endless talk of 'care' yet little compassion. We are all dependent on someone, but some people can only make changes when they are sure of your kindness towards them.

Often, new patients would come into my office in a state of complete despair. Jennifer was furious. 'I don't know why I'm here. You can't help me. My mother is sitting out there, you can go and ask her. She followed me here to make sure that I came.'

I put my notes on the floor beside me and gently replied, 'You don't have to tell me anything . . . but your GP thought I might be able to help, so that's why he wrote to me.'

'Can you? Nobody knows what's wrong with me. The doctor at the other hospital has suddenly said he won't treat me any more.'

She burst into tears. 'I've seen that bloody bastard for ages, and he just told me to get lost . . . Can you help? I bet you can't. I think I'm beyond help.'

'I don't know.' Being honest is kinder than superficiality and pretence. I was telling the truth. I was also worried. Behind the bravado she sounded quite hopeless. She snorted but grabbed a tissue from the box that I offered her, so I continued slowly. 'It will mean telling me what's been going on . . . It must be very upsetting . . . coming all the way here to see someone else. Having to go through it all again. Do you think we might try?'

There was a pause, then 'Okay,' she nodded hesitantly.

I didn't pick up the notes, but left them in the floor, my focus on her. 'Tell me what's been happening to you?'

Jennifer's last consultant had told her he thought she might have an eating disorder and that she needed specialist treatment. She disagreed. An argument ensued and he had discharged her from his care with the statement, in his letter, that she needed to 'learn to take more responsibility for herself'. This wasn't the first time this had happened to her, and it almost seemed Jennifer was determined to prove that I wasn't going to be willing to see her either. Sometimes that is how it is. I can remember practically inviting the therapist who helped me the most, to confirm my worst fears about myself – by being obnoxious to him at times, but he never rejected me. A person can reach a point where it's impossible to find the emotional energy to deal with anything other than self-protection and survival. The act of telling others how we feel inside and risking their rejection when we are at our most vulnerable, is too frightening.

'You don't have to say any more if you don't want to,' I said quietly. Telling people to try harder is not kind, it's inhumane. 'But maybe I can try and understand?'

By listening and showing that you care, you help a person invest in a more fulfilling relationship with the world. There is too much talk about encouraging people to be responsible for themselves, but not enough compassion for others or ourselves.

I'm starting to explore in my writing what I love, and hate, about the memories, thoughts and feelings that the idea of 'kindness' summons up. Maybe that is a way forward.

This morning, Katie the errant cat from last year reappeared on the windowsill in front of my desk. She returned to the garden a couple of weeks ago and has been coming three times a day and more for food. Last week I buried worming tablets in her food which she inhaled as rapidly as ever. Her ambivalence about me seems to be shifting slightly. She allows me to stroke her head as she paces about at the threshold and rewards me by purring loudly.

My life would be inestimably improved if I could find some respite from the controller in my brain.

Pushing myself to walk to my favourite vantage point, the seat above the harbour in Stromness. It is too damp to sit down, and today's precipitation is poised somewhere between fine, gentle rain and mist. I watch the Hamnavoe in the Sound, and her small sibling, Graemsay, come and go from Hoy. Each day they ply the Northern waters in and out of the harbour. When the seas are choppy, they may miss a day or two, but the boats always return to their daily schedule, even if the going can be a little rough for the passengers. The children from North Hoy come to school in Stromness every day on the ferry. What an extraordinary start and finish to the day that would be, except in stormy weather.

Gathering my coat around me against the cold wind, I watch a fishing vessel silhouetted against the sky, close my eyes, breathe gently, feel the raindrops on my skin and focus on the sounds of the wind, the soaring gulls and the waves as they lap against the shore and, for a few precious minutes, time is suspended.

CHAPTER 6

In sickness and in health

Orkney is sliding from spring into summer all around me. Back in the field now with their calves, the cows stare at me when I go outside. No respecters of boundaries, they stretch over the fence to sample the greener grass of our lawn. We are sleeping in the attic in the spare bed, which the delivery men had such difficulty getting up the narrow and steep staircase.

'Don't reckon you'll ever get that down these stairs again without sawing it in two,' one of them cheerfully informed me.

We are up here while downstairs is being decorated. The front and side windows have all been replaced and now John is busy painting the walls. My desk is covered in a dust sheet. The attic ceiling slopes down low on each side so you can only stand upright in the centre of the room. 'I love it up here, it's like being in a tent!' he says. We take pleasure in childish things.

Each morning this week, we have had hares in the garden. Sometimes two or three, munching away on the wildflowers. 'It's the dandelions they like,' Bob tells me. They treat our corner of the field like a delicatessen, but when the grass has been cut back, they disappear for a while. Fortunately, they don't take the purple orchids sticking up here and there out of the lawn, and Bob skilfully skirts around them with the mower.

Despite all this activity, and life going on around us, something feels wrong. I sleep for nine hours but wake with no sense of being refreshed, just a persisting somnolence. When I do manage to get into gear, I feel too tired to go out, and just want to sleep on the sofa.

Meanwhile, John is preoccupied with the sound of house sparrows, who have hatched their chicks this year in a gap between the end wall of the house and the roof. He has been outside watching them take turns to visit the nest.

'Can't you hear them?' he asks. 'Aren't they bothering you?'

'No, I can't hear anything.' There are some advantages to the deafness that comes with increasing age. High-pitched sounds are lost. The birds could come and go all day and never disturb my sleep.

He tries to push me to go out for a walk. 'Exercise would help you know . . . and some fresh air.'

As one of those people who resists pressure with an equal and opposing force I reply, 'I'm too tired. Anyway, I've still got some work to do.' It is warm and sunny outside, a perfect day to go out, but I just want to lie down on the sofa.

'You haven't really retired, have you?'

He gets annoyed because he cares, but I get irritated and we argue. 'I'm worried about me too. You go on your own. I will feel better later.'

Depression and anxiety are not only experienced in the mind, but in the body too. When illness involves our bodies, it has an impact on our minds – and vice versa. They are intimately related.

Since the day of being diagnosed with kidney disease I have monitored my body closely, observing how aches and pains shift mysteriously from one joint to another. How my heart misses a beat or speeds up more often than it used to. How the pain that I woke with in my right arm (which I have self-diagnosed as tennis elbow) has increased in intensity as the small hand has moved around the kitchen clock ... probably because I've been thinking about it all the time. The more I dwell on it, the worse it becomes. *Is it arthritis?* I worry much more about my health these days.

Years ago, I remember seeing in my clinic a middle-aged man, Jim, who was worried about pains all over his body, which he had experienced for many years. He'd had multiple investigations, which revealed nothing much, and he'd been told that he had 'medically unexplained symptoms'.[7] We sat down with his case notes and discussed the tests that had been carried out across different departments at the hospital. Whatever the cause, his quality of life was affected, and I hoped we could improve on that. Confined to bed for much of the time, he found it hard to be active and was angry and exasperated with the medical profession. As we turned the pages of his case notes he asked questions, and I tried to answer.

'So "at the top of the normal range" it says there,' pointing to a particular blood result, 'that's not good then is it? I mean it's high, isn't it?'

'It's still within normal limits.' We looked through previous pages for comparisons, which seemed to relieve him, but after about half an hour he fell silent, looking down at his hands and flexing his fingers as though testing their range of movement.

'All these tests and scans . . . they've never checked me out here, have they?' he said pointing to his left flank. 'That's where the pain is worst at the moment.'

I didn't know how to reply. Just about every part of Jim's body had been thoroughly investigated.

Yet now, with persistent discomfort in my left flank, I know how he felt. I was constantly checking and prodding and trying to reassure myself, but it was only when my scan results were explained to me at the kidney clinic, that I realised the pains had gone. I was sure they had told me the kidney on that side was enlarged, but it wasn't, and the pains were worse when my mood was low. By dwelling on aches that I usually would have put down to slumping on the sofa for too long, I magnified their intensity.

This time however, I'm sure it is not just my imagination. I've had persistent bladder symptoms for the last couple of years, but nothing was found until, a month ago, I started to pee blood red urine.

'There must be an infection!' I insisted to my GP.

'They can't find one. It might possibly be that one of your kidney cysts has burst and caused the bleeding, but that is usually painful.' At the clinic they were equally unsure what was going on. 'You will have to come back for more tests.'

Then the bleeding stopped as suddenly as it had begun. I had not imagined it and am due for more tests when we return south next week.

People with kidney disease are more likely to be depressed and anxious and it's very similar for all types of chronic illness.

When I was still a doctor, Mavis, a patient of mine with 'chronic obstructive airways disease' had struggled to tell me what she was still able to enjoy doing despite her breathlessness.

It wasn't difficult to see why Mavis was finding everyday life more difficult than ever even though her lung function was better than would have been predicted from how she was coping. Her daughter seemed relentlessly negative, focussing only on problems her mother's illness caused.

'We can't take her on holiday. It's too embarrassing for her when she coughs up all that vile stuff at the dining table. She's breathless too and gets upset because she can't keep up when we go out.' She suddenly turned to her mother, 'I'm sorry Mum, but that's how it is isn't it?'

Mavis nodded. It must have sounded as if her active life was over.

Exhausted now, I sometimes wonder if I will soon go to sleep forever. In guided meditation I even resent the instructions to feel compassionate and caring. *I've spent my life caring for others. What about me?* Trapped in a paradoxical loop, I work too hard to achieve a sense of peace.

'Just after you gave up work,' says John, 'I thought the person I married was back, but now I only get glimpses of her, and I miss her.' He has told me this so many times. 'You still want to be the best, to achieve that success, to please your father . . . ' his voice tails off.

A sharp pain in my chest is followed by a tear running down my cheek. He is right, and I am terribly afraid of losing him. 'Do you still love me?' I ask.

'Of course, I do! Look, I know you are worried about your kidneys,' he hugs me and whispers, 'I am too. I try not to show it, but I am.'

The difference between the depression and my kidney disease is that if depression were to kill me it would be because I wanted it to. Even though I know rationally, as a psychiatrist, that my choice would be strongly influenced by my mental state at the time. Like many doctors, I am prone to think I can cheat fate and carry on forever.

When I was a medical student in Edinburgh, we gathered around the bed of a patient, a heavy smoker, who was breathless and coughing up blood. The surgeon gave her his usual stern ticking off about the dangers of cigarettes, and we trooped back to the doctor's office where he took the patient's chest x-ray out of the envelope and pushed it up onto the lightbox on the wall. 'Look at the mass there,' he said, pointing to a dense shadow in the left lung, 'almost certainly a carcinoma,' and took a packet of Senior Service out of the pocket of his white coat, puffing away as we discussed the prognosis.

About the same time, sitting in the McEwan Hall in Edinburgh and feeling the glands in my neck whilst sitting a written examination on pathology, I tried to convince myself that slightly enlarged lumps weren't the first sign of Hodgkin's Disease. I went to see my GP.

'So, what are you studying at the moment?' he asked, 'Let me guess . . . I think I know what it is this month.'

Medical students have always alternated between being sure they have every disease they learn about and complete denial of their own susceptibility. Like the surgeon who smoked, doctors can maintain a peculiar belief in their own immortality. As if knowing about disease not only gives you power over it but also makes you immune. This is one of the excuses we whisper to ourselves while we fail to take care of our own health.

*

Depression brings changes to our lives, and we often have to make further changes because of it, but some things cannot be changed. We must find ways of living with them.

Paul Gilbert talks about three different systems that operate in our brains, which illustrate how I try to manage my emotions. My 'threat and self-protection system' is highly sensitive. I can be a fearful, nervous girl, expecting to be 'found out'. Another part of me, which Gilbert labels the 'incentive and resource seeking system', is a striving perfectionist desperate to prove herself, to not only succeed but to be the best. Not only is this exactly what the fearful girl most dreads, the expected pleasure at winning is never enough, and the fear of failure can lead to the paralysis of relentless rumination – *should I try or not*? I also want what Gilbert calls the 'soothing-contentment system', that part of our brain that helps us to feel more peaceful and balanced, to kick in as it does after a period of calm meditation, but I have always pushed myself harder and harder, so the calm feelings melt away too soon. I may have transferred the perfectionist attitude of my working years to my plans for retirement.

As a group, medics score high on perfectionism. It's one of the things we talk about when I'm asked to speak to medical students about mental health and I've treated students and doctors, both young and old, during my career.

A student, Amy, who came up to me at the end of a lecture told me, 'I'm worried that I've damaged my brain.' There wasn't any evidence for this. Her GP had already tried hard to reassure her, but she didn't believe him. 'I think it's going to kill me. My brain is dying, because I've been working so hard and not getting any sleep.' She was very distressed.

Amy told a familiar story. She had been one of the brightest students in her school, but on arrival at university found herself in a class full of stars, who all worked hard. Amy's response was to work even harder, going to great lengths to try and cover everything in great depth – setting herself unachievable goals. I'd been there too. After we had talked further, I explained, 'I think you are seriously depressed, and you need to take some time away from studies and get some help.' Her mood was very low, and the ideas about her brain being damaged sounded rather like the kind of 'hypochondriacal delusions' – abnormal beliefs about health and illness, that are seen in very severe depression, so I arranged for her to be seen urgently.

Despite the stresses of the job, we carry on, not only being perfectionists but very competitive too. It's hard to step away from competition that feeds your own sense of self-worth, being good at *something*. So, when we retire, we may carry on competing – with ourselves. Setting goals for things we want to achieve, studying again, even sitting more examinations – because that is what we have always done to feel good, however much we hate it. Or we don't give up the job. A good friend of mine who has suffered serious physical illness, and been depressed too, says he cannot retire because, 'I don't know what else I could do.'

Recovering from depression means getting to know who we really are and what we want from life, and not trying to please other people, even if that means annoying them. During therapy we may glimpse a new, more real and authentic version of ourselves. Someone who can do things that the 'old' version would never have dared to try. At another of life's crossroads we have a choice: turn off this track and take the uphill road to explore what lies in the valley beyond that mountain ahead, or carry on along the same relentless road.

Katie, meanwhile, has been striving to achieve her goal of eating as much as possible. She has been back here two or three times a day since our return, most days pawing at the back window or sitting on the front sill with an imploring gaze. She seems hungrier than ever – and broader too.

'Do you think she might be pregnant?' I ask John, 'I wormed her last time, but she is still ravenous.'

'She's beginning to look like one of those "wide loads" you see on the motorway.'

This last few days she has started to come in and eat from the kitchen counter, retreating through the back window at any sign of encouragement. She teases me by rolling around on the flagstones by the front door, always just out of reach – rather like my sense of well-being. I think she's wary of getting too close, but we are leaving tomorrow morning on the early ferry and how will she manage for food?

Next day in the silver light of dawn I watch for Katie as we drive up the lane towards Stromness, but there is no sign.

More than two months have gone by since then, and my heart feels strangely lighter than it has done for months. I'm slouching on my favourite sofa, which is really a chaise longue (every psychiatrist should have one), and John is sitting across from me, listening as I explain why I arrived back in Orkney over an hour later than expected.

'I couldn't call. By the time we knew that we were heading towards a boat in distress I couldn't get a phone signal.'

Twenty minutes out of Scrabster I was pondering whether to look for somewhere in the bar to stretch out as that usually helps me feel less seasick. When the captain's voice came over the tannoy, I was wondering if eating my usual fish and chips on the boat had been such a good idea.

'*We are heading directly north.*'

'We were going to the aid of a yacht that was taking on water,' I explain to John, 'When we got there, the Stromness lifeboat was arriving from the opposite direction. One of the crew jumped on board and started to pump out the water, but we hung around for a while to make sure everything was OK.'

Everyone on the ferry had watched as the volunteer life-boatman took command, balancing nimbly on the gunwales of the tiny yacht, while the two people aboard stood at the stern with their arms around each other.

'I am so pleased to be back here with you.' I say and reach out to hold his hand.

'I'm relieved,' he tells me, 'and Katie is fine too, you will be delighted to know.'

She had started visiting Mary at the farm after we left the island and took her new-born kittens there too. She must have given birth just as soon as we had departed. 'They've all been rehomed by Cats' Protection,' John says, 'Even Katie.' Ambivalent about being in a permanent relationship with humans, she will be fine as long as she has a barn to retreat into.

In Yorkshire, John came with me to see my psychiatrist because I thought his contribution might be helpful. I also wanted his support, wondering if I was on too much medica-tion. Why was I sleeping all the time? Since the last serious relapse, I'd been on two different antidepressants and had difficulty finding the right words – a major problem for a writer.

'Is there any chance I might come off the buproprion?' I asked. It had helped enormously when I was unwell, but now ... Like most people on tablets I wanted to stop taking them.

'And replace it with something else?'

'Try without?'

'You know the advice is to stay on what gets you well and of course ...' I knew exactly what he was going to say, 'cognitive difficulties could be explained by depression.'

The problem was that nothing kept me completely well, so when I relapsed I tended to end up on more medication each time – but that was what I was thinking. It's a conversation I'd been through with my own patients many times. On several different pills you wonder what you would be like taking fewer, but the only way forwards was to up the dosage, not clean the blackboard and start again. My symptoms could be explained by depression, but there were other possibilities.

'I think everything really started after I went for the investigations,' I say this evening. John and I have only been apart for a month but it feels more like a year. Since getting back I've had a desire to drink tea, mug after mug. There is never any tea like the tea you drink at home.

'How are you now? Have you got any physical symptoms at all?' he asks.

'None at all.'

The Hallamshire hospital in Sheffield is a perfect example of a neo-Stalinist public building from the second half of the twentieth century: massive, anonymous, and without character. Many years ago, I had an office there, with no external windows and only artificial light. I never knew what weather to expect when I left in the evening. It was a lonely place to work – with a rumoured high suicide rate among junior doctors who rarely met. The last time I had been there was for a Magnetic Resonance Image (MRI) scan, a willing volunteer in a research project, or that is what the Professor of Nephrology told me. Lying on my back, wearing earmuffs, I listened to the disjointed clangs, clicks and buzzing of the scanner as it constructed a detailed image of my abdomen. The noises vibrated through my body and seemed, in my mind, to focus and pull on my wedding ring, the single piece of metal I was allowed to retain, even though I knew it wasn't magnetic.

A disembodied voice instructed me to 'breathe in... breathe out ... breathe in again and hold your breath. Once more ... breathe in ... breathe ... breathe in again and hold your breath.' The voice played a remorseless game with me.

Maybe it was because I knew what to expect this time, but the usual scans and endoscopic examination were over very quickly. Afterwards I found my way to the cafeteria where I could have drunk something much stronger but settled for lemonade. Once, I would have felt at ease here, the surgical staff sitting at a table in their blue scrubs, the unappetizing food and the constant buzz of conversation. Now, I had no desire to return to medical life, but then the unexpected happened and, within a week, I was back in hospital as a patient.

Sitting together on the sofa this evening in Orkney, several weeks later, I don't think I have realised how much it has all affected John. It is getting late, but the summer sun remains above the horizon, casting a golden light over the fields. In Brazil, which straddles the equator, night comes suddenly but in the northern latitudes of Orkney the summer gloaming lasts for hours. We hold hands and remember what happened, talking our way through it, making sense of it in our own fashion. A tractor passes along the road, a farmer working late. The scent of recently mown grass after Bob has cut the lawn. The hares remain in the field and, in summer, it is impossible to imagine the wind and rain of an Orkney winter. It feels as if nothing will ever change but, at the back of your mind, you know it will. The storms will return again. It feels wrong to spoil the moment by recalling the recent past, but we need to talk about it. John perhaps more than me. We have been apart for a while.

'I have never ever seen you look so ill as you did that night you went into hospital,' he says. 'It felt like I was losing you, it was terrible,' he pauses, 'but when I met the doctor who saw you the second time, I could see you were in good hands.'

It began in the middle of Sunday night as a pain in my left side, then I started to vomit. After going through the routine questions with the person at the emergency phone-line (just my luck to get sick on a Bank Holiday) I was sent to the Emergency Department at our local hospital in Yorkshire. The Casualty Officer took me through his deliberations: 'Pain and some renal angle tenderness, recent invasive investigation, and a very slight rise in temperature but ...'

Each symptom might, or might not, be important, and I had no other signs of infection. However, my kidneys were slowly turning into something like Swiss cheese. Perhaps I really had been bleeding intermittently into one of their many holes. He sent me home with a supply of codeine. 'Come back immediately if you feel any worse ...'

Thirty-six hours later I was back in severe pain, incoherent, vomiting and shaking uncontrollably as the rigors, the attacks of shivering that accompany a sudden rise in temperature, took hold. 'Take me back to the hospital now, please,' I said to John just before bedtime. 'I feel like I'm dying.' Any longer and I might have been.

They took me straight into a cubicle to find that my blood pressure was falling, and my metabolism going awry. A second doctor diagnosed sepsis in need of urgent treatment. Within minutes I was catheterised and had a drip in each arm.

The septicaemia, meaning bacteria in my bloodstream in considerable numbers, sent me into a state bordering on delirium. I knew that I was in a hospital ward, and that it was the elderly unit as that was the only place a bed was available, but I was convinced there was an underground railway station at my end of the four-bedded ward where, below me to the right, beneath the window, waiting for trains to arrive and leave from the platform, people were talking. Every few hours they came to inject me with antibiotics and, at some point, I got into a debate with the poor junior doctor about whether it was correct to release the tourniquet before or after taking the needle out as she pushed at my remaining veins for more blood. She was trying to see what bugs my blood would grow in her culture bottles.

'You always take the tourniquet off first, don't you? That's odd,' I rambled on, 'because I'm sure I always took the needle out first, before I loosened the tourniquet. I've been lying here thinking about it, trying to work it out.'

After she melted into the darkness, I ruminated feverishly about whether that had or had not been my routine practice and decided it probably hadn't after all. The effect of septicaemia on my brain resembled alcohol, impairing my judgment and loosening my tongue.

The ward had a brutal daily regimen. Each morning I was expected by the night staff to get out of bed and sit in a chair with no pillow for two hours, even though I was unable to support my own weight, while I waited for the day staff to 'come and do the beds'. After a couple of days, I rebelled and crawled back onto the bare mattress where I fell asleep on the sticky plastic sheeting, but they didn't come any sooner and left me until last. I heard the nurses refer to the lady in the next bed, who was barely conscious, as a 'bed-blocker' and am certain that wasn't a figment of my delirium. I refused to get up at 6.30 a.m. and my increasingly stained sheets were left unchanged for 3 days while the dressing on one of the tubes I had in each arm began to discolour and smell. Neither the nurses nor the ever-changing doctors introduced themselves and I couldn't read their name badges as I didn't have my glasses with me. I gradually learned which nurses to ask if I wanted something, and which would ignore me or get impatient.

One evening, one of the kinder nurses whispered, 'I've been a patient too, I know what it's like when no-one listens to you or tells you anything.' I could have hugged her for saying that.

'That ward that you were on at first was terrible.'

It is getting late, but I don't feel ready to sleep. I still need to talk to John. To touch his face, hold his hands, and be here with him again. I cannot help but grimace at the memory.

'I told you about when I pressed the call bell and no-one came.'

I had been in severe pain. A half hour went by and I began to wonder how long it would be before anyone came to check on our ward. That was the point when I could fully understand how a person might want to break the window and leap into the comforting darkness, as one of my own patients did many years ago. She told me, much later after recovering from her injuries, how no-one took seriously how unwell she felt. Some of the staff made fun of her too. I suspected this was because her case notes mentioned 'personality disorder'.

'They seemed to think I was just a nuisance and it was all my own fault for being there after taking an overdose. I couldn't take any more, so I jumped.'

Looking at the thin pane of glass separating me from the night sky, I considered it. Shortly after that a staff nurse arrived. 'What's the matter?' she asked.

Immediately I felt ashamed for my distress, although I know now that I shouldn't have. When I wrote to the Chief Executive afterwards, he asked me if I wanted to make a complaint about how the ward was run. I replied that I didn't, I simply wanted something to change. As a junior doctor I learned how many people get depressed, despondent and even suicidal in an acute hospital unit. How we are feeling in our spirits plays an important part in how we cope with serious physical illnesses. What we expect to happen to us has a bearing on what actually does, (although I'm not suggesting you can simply think yourself better) and if we are feeling down a good conversation with a nurse can help us feel much more hopeful.

After a few days one of the senior nurses came into the room to chat and giggle with some of the nursing assistants. The same ones who, since finding out I was a psychiatrist, had been teasing me about it in a way which amused them ('Go on then, analyse us, bet you can'). They reminded me of school bullies. I couldn't hear much of what was said as I wasn't wearing my hearing aid. Picking up her paperwork after a cursory glance at each of us patients, as though we were invisible, she left and I had a sudden and painful premonition of my future as a frail elderly person approaching death, in this room. Yet each of the four of us in those beds, despite our infirmities, was still breathing, dreaming and present not only in our own conscious lives but those of our families, even if our hopes and dreams were marginal to the lives of our temporary carers. Unable to tell the difference between dreams and reality, I experienced nightmares.

Later, feeling human again, I had a painful yearning for the purple hills of Hoy as viewed from my desk. The last time I was there, out of season, I visited the shore at Rackwick, on the west coast overlooking the Atlantic. Where a river winds its way across a heather swathed valley beneath those magnificent red sandstone cliffs towards the sea, a place haunted by the ghosts of crofters. This bay, near the Old Man, was the first part of Orkney that I saw all those years ago. Entirely alone, by the stone wall of a bothy, looking up at the washing lines of the few houses that are inhabited all year round, I wondered if I could manage the isolation.

Rackwick is where the composer, Peter Maxwell Davies, lived for many years. Lying in bed I could see, with my mind's eye, the cliffs, the boulder strewn bay and the yellow strand of the beach at low tide. Did the waves crashing on the shore below his home inspire his music? I remembered the painting of Rackwick on my wall and knew without doubt that I would see it again.

Halfway through my stay, I was transferred to another ward.

'Gosh, what have you got in your arm?' the senior nurse who greeted me took one look at the sight of the stained dressing around the tube hanging from my wrist. 'When was that last changed? Get into bed and I'll see to that straight away.'

This was a surgical ward, and it soon filled completely with some very unwell people. Each nurse introduced themselves with 'Hello my name is . . . '[8] and I became visible again as a person who was sick and in need of care and assistance. Each day my bed was remade, and I was able to get back into it if I needed, as I was still exhausted. It felt as though I had been moved to a different hospital, not just to another floor.

John had been relieved when they moved me, 'That's when I could see the end of the tunnel,' he said. 'Every day I parked in that car park, came up to see you, and went home and ate something although I wasn't hungry. I just had to keep myself going.'

'I finally asked you to bring some fruit and yoghurt in for me,' I replied. It was all that I could eat. 'The food inside was inedible.'

'Yes,' he laughs. 'That was a very positive sign!'

My appetite is back to normal now. I feel like starting to cook again. 'There was a nurse on the ward, you know, who had the same problem as I do.' I don't think I had told him at the time, so I tell him now.

I was still being treated for the infection in my kidney, which had caused the sepsis, when one of the nurses said. 'I've got the same diagnosis that you have, polycystic kidneys. I had very high blood pressure, that's how they found it. I'm okay now, really I'm fine.'

We were both under the care of the same consultant, and somehow seeing her working filled me with hope. At the same time, I worried that the infection might have hastened the speed at which my kidney function was deteriorating. I still don't know the answer to this. Frequent infections are not a good sign but, as I regained both strength and interest in the world beyond the ward window, a change began in my view of the future. I was lucky to be alive. Fast access to the right treatment is crucial in sepsis. John had taken me back to the hospital at the right time. If we had waited until morning, I would have been even more ill. Now, I have a sense of a door opening into a second chance at the future. How I am going to spend the rest of this life I've been given? I don't want to feel like a passive victim of my health problems. I cannot expect never to be depressed again at some point but I'm going to find a way to have a better life despite that.

I think once more of Mavis, the lady with the chest problems, and her daughter whom I met many years ago in Salford. I knew she had been a publican and asked her, 'What was it like, running a pub around here before they built all the tower blocks? Do you remember?'

'Yes, of course I do!' Over the next few minutes she changed from the timid mother who waited for her daughter to answer for her, to a person who had a story to tell. Between spasms of coughing, she reminisced about all the people who used to come into the pub. She had a reputation for running a respectable bar and wasn't afraid to deal with drunks who wouldn't leave.

'You were a bit of a tough one, weren't you, Mum?' her daughter put in. In their shared smile I could see clearly the mutual affection that had been absent earlier.

'What else can you still do despite the breathlessness?' I asked.

I suspected nobody ever spoke any more about all the things she had achieved in her life and asked her what she still was able to enjoy. They just reminded her what she couldn't. I wanted to help her both remember her past but still believe in a future. The stories or 'narratives' that we tell about ourselves when we are sick are very powerful. Everyone wants to hear about the stories in which we get sick, have our treatment and get back to our old self again, but there are also those other less cheerful stories where life doesn't improve. Stories about how difficult life can be when bad things happen still need to be told. I tried to help Mavis remember the person she had been before she became ill. Someone who was still inside her, but slowly being forgotten even by Mavis herself.

I too can't get back to the person I used to be, and so dislike how professionals talk about you being on your 'recovery journey'. It can feel like you are being told you must reach your destination and 'get well' whatever is happening to you. However, I have been on a journey of sorts for a long time, a quest to better understand myself, and I am in the driving seat. Only me, not my doctor or anyone else.

I've already made an important decision, having stopped taking one of two antidepressants. That's two now instead of four pills. I know the medication should have been tapered off slowly. The withdrawal symptoms are very real.

One morning when I was sitting up in bed, the staff nurse came around to unlock the drawer next to my bed and give me my medication: antibiotics, thyroxine, vitamins and these depression pills. Three small white tablets, two huge grey and white capsules, a blue and white capsule and two big white pills in a plastic container.

'I'm going to stop the big white one,' I said. 'The buproprion.'

'Really? Can you do that? I thought you were supposed to be on them. You were before you came in here. Don't they stop you . . . ?'

'I spoke to my doctor on the phone.' I had indeed. His secretary got the message to him and he called me back. 'I'm at the Isle of Wight Rock Festival,' he had shouted above what sounded like heavy metal. Was I being a typically difficult doctor-patient by bothering him? I had wanted to stop them before, the last time I saw him, and he had persuaded me not to.

'Okay,' he had said, 'Go ahead. You can always go back on them if needed.'

'Well, we don't want you to go funny on us,' the nurse said, giving me even more of a suspicious look than she had when she had said 'depression pills.'

Lying in a bed with a health professional standing next to you, you need to be aware of who holds the cards, so I bit my tongue. I also didn't seem to need the antihypertensives either, my blood pressure was still rock bottom. Fewer tablets: I felt better just for that. In the end, any symptoms of withdrawal from the antidepressants were masked by everything else that was still playing havoc with my metabolism.

A few days later my two week stay in hospital ended. Dressed for the first time since entering the Emergency Department, my dress hung loosely from my shoulders. I had lost weight. In the open air the mild breeze reminded me that it was summer. 'Steps here,' John warned. Lifting my feet was an effort but I ascended the short staircase with care and a few paces later we arrived at the car.

'I've really missed you.' He touched my hands and clasped my knees as we drove towards the motorway junction. Shop windows flashed by. Traffic lights. I remembered the road. I used to travel to work along it.

'I'm really pleased I'm still here,' I said, and I meant it.

This evening, once more in the glow of the Orkney summer night, I feel at peace for the first time in weeks. With the most important person in my life beside me the future seems less of a challenge. I don't have to face it alone.

CHAPTER 7

True North

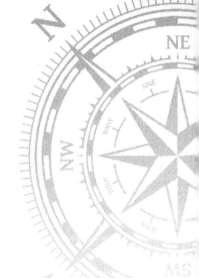

Rosie was a striking young woman with pale skin and long red hair, about the same age as me, whom I met on the ferry, the St Ola, coming into Stromness in 1974. Today, as John and I walk through the streets of Stromness past the Town Hall, a converted church that once doubled as a Youth Hostel in the summer months, I find myself thinking of her. Rosie and I both stayed there.

'I did too,' says the woman who runs the knitwear shop as John sorts through pullovers.

'It was girls on the stage and boys in the main hall, on the other side of a curtain, and they drew a little Viking blowing a horn on my YHA card before I left.' They didn't use an official stamp. I still have that membership card.

'I came back for good,' she tells me.

Have I?

A significant part of recovery is about re-evaluating moments in life that have been important to you and working out how you feel about them now. Each moment is encapsulated in your memories of a place.

Only a couple of weeks after I came out of hospital, we were travelling north again, to Edinburgh. This time the journey was more stressful than usual. I had only just begun to recover from sepsis. John turned to me.

'How are you feeling? Let me know when you want to stop.'

'I'm okay, really.'

'You aren't in any pain?'

There was some in my left side again, over my kidney. I could hear in his voice how concerned he still was about me. I was worried too. It was almost the end of June. In another couple of weeks, I was supposed to be flying to Canada for a journey that had been planned for a year and would now separate us for almost a month.

'I just feel very tired. I might nod off for a while.'

I can sleep anywhere, even the front of a Volkswagen Golf with the seat upright. On waking though, the accompanying snort can be loud and embarrassing, especially on aeroplanes. This time the physical exhaustion was worse than ever.

That the A1M leads to Scotland is its only saving grace and I never tire of seeing the road signs that simply say 'To the North' – no fussy towns or cities added to the big metal boards.

'I'm not sure if I'll manage without the "sat nav",' he warned, his nickname for a combination of me and the road map. I usually love finding my way around a road atlas but couldn't summon up any enthusiasm. The evil controller had sneaked into my head and moved around the chess pieces while reminding me that I didn't know how to play.

'Remember I have no sense of direction without you,' he said as I drifted into stupor.

I woke as we approached Hadrian's Wall, passing invisibly through a wide gap in the Roman frontier marked by a great stone which proclaims England on one side, and Scotland on the other.

Rosie with the red hair had told me that she was going to study art in Edinburgh, where I was, then, just about to begin medicine. Only a few months after we met in Orkney, I bumped into her on Laurieston Place near the Art School.

'Hello, how are you?' I asked. 'Do you remember me?'

'Of course, I do! I'm fine, doing well. How are you?'

She was a familiar and friendly face when I was feeling very lonely, but I was too shy to stay in touch.

Having arrived in Edinburgh as a green eighteen-year-old from the east of England, only a couple of months after that first visit to Orkney, I did a great deal of my growing up there. I have blood ties to Scotland, but they come from the soot-grey towns of North Lanarkshire, not the shortbread tin beauty of Edinburgh. I didn't fit in with the middle-class natives like my first husband, whose grandmother not only went to Cramond Kirk, but had an account at Jenners on Princes Street. Many of the other English students were Oxbridge rejects, like me, but from families that went to the 'continent' for holidays, and regularly drank wine with dinner. I didn't fit in with them either, being the only member of my extended family to go to university or leave the country for something other than to go to war. My parents would have a glass of Cyprus cream sherry on special occasions.

It wasn't long before I discovered that Edinburgh was

simply better than the West of Scotland at hiding its ugliness and poverty under fancy skirts: in the tower blocks of Wester Hailes and tenements of West Pilton and Craigmillar, well away from the city centre. Some of our teachers who were from the South of England had difficulty understanding a broad Edinburgh accent. 'Can anyone help me here?' I remember a posh young chest physician turning to ask the group of students around the bed. A man in his fifties from West Granton, who looked twenty years older than his date of birth suggested, was trying to explain how he couldn't get his breath.

Last time I took John on an evening stroll around the University and bored him with reminiscences that each building and street corner whispered to me. For decades I avoided Edinburgh through fear of encountering ghosts from the past but, now, after forty years, I found myself enjoying the cobbled streets and telling John embarrassing tales of student days. Falling off the high kerb in the High Street on a drunken three-legged pub crawl and being unable to walk the next day. Trying, and failing, to get up Arthur's Seat on Mayday to wash my face in the morning dew (it was supposed to make you beautiful) because of my inability to rise early – even oversleeping on the morning of our only lecture on sleep. Lying on the grass in the sunshine, in George Square, the day the results of Finals were pinned to the door of the Old Medical School, unable to believe I had passed.

As John and I walked past the old Royal Infirmary, boarded up for conversion into luxury flats, I told him about standing proudly outside the main entrance, under the clock, for the traditional group photograph of house officers not long before leaving the city for good – part of a long list of famous alumni from Charles Darwin to Arthur Conan Doyle. We were only a short distance from where I had spoken to Rosie a few years before.

With inexplicable anxiety about leaving an unhappy family, I failed to manage my problems with mood and married far too young. An ambivalent medical student, and for many years an ambivalent doctor, I never felt I belonged anywhere.

We are walking the boggy track along the West Mainland coast towards Yesnaby Castle, one of Orkney's great sea stacks. Forged over millennia from sedimentary layers, it once formed part of an arch connecting to the angular cliffs. Now, the arch having collapsed into the sea, it stands precariously on two narrow columns of stone. John has always been entranced by Yesnaby. He returns here time after time to photograph it in every season when the state of the sea changes from rough to calm and the sky from black to blue. Tourists rarely stray beyond the end of road and buildings left over from the second world war. Strike out either North or South and you find deep peace and quiet.

'I love the sense of escaping from everything here,' he says, 'it's so far away, I feel distant from everything going on at home.'

When he is here, he can't respond to his mother by getting in the car and driving over, as he has done to almost every family summons over the last couple of decades. A phone call has to be sufficient, and now there are others more directly involved in caring.

He has been in Orkney for a month or so while I was in Canada, and there is always pressure on him to return to Yorkshire. 'I have to go and take care of Mum's garden,' he says. 'The lawn needs mowing, and the hedges will have grown in the last month.'

'How do you feel about moving here permanently?' We talked for years about eventually moving to Scotland, but it seemed always to be in the future. 'It's more than escape for me,' I say, 'It feels like home now.'

Now I'm back from my travels he must be getting bored hearing about them: my trip to Gwaii Haanas, the special place to which I had long wanted to return. Every time I look at the small collection of photographs taken during the journey I am transported there again.

Sitting, one morning, on the covered porch of my wooden 'lodge', floating a few yards from dry land, I watched falling raindrops form tiny ripples on the otherwise mirror-like surface of the inlet. Grey-green slopes rose from the water's edge. Two bald eagles soared between the tops of the spruce trees. I'd been learning the names of the vegetation and wildlife from our guide and thinking how much richer my experience of Orkney would be if I could do the same. The rigid inflatable Zodiac we had been travelling in was docked nearby. Soon we would be setting off again, but for a few minutes I could enjoy the silence, the faint pine perfume of the forest and the soft morning light. With all my senses engaged I was at peace.

The writer Richard Mabey characterised being 'healed' as not so much being taken out of yourself by nature, but rather by the wild outdoors entering your mind and reigniting your imagination. Just as it does when I'm standing outside my front door in Orkney, looking down the valley and watching the towering silver-grey clouds at the leading edge of a weather front advancing, as they usually do, from the South West. Exposure to natural spaces is immensely beneficial to us in all kinds of ways. Perhaps there is some evolutionary explanation, but a sense of somewhere as 'my place', a spiritual home however temporary, seems very important to me.

The trip was meant to be not only a return to Gwaii Haanas after sixteen years, but also an attempt at regaining the sense of freedom and self-possession I had achieved as a solitary traveller in Scotland. I first heard about Haida Gwaii more than thirty years ago when flicking through a copy of *National Geographic* and saw Canadian First Nations People, the Haida, linking arms in front of huge logging trucks, trying to prevent the destruction of their islands.

Like the native inhabitants of the Northern Isles, the Haida are physically tough and fiercely proud. On my first visit, in the small town of Masset, I drank coffee not in Starbucks but in the aptly named *HaidaBucks*. Revisiting the totem poles and once more experiencing the presence of the Great Spirit in the rainforest would be a special kind of medicine for my soul.

The problem was that I did not plan on being seriously ill a month before the journey and far from peak fitness, which achieves only foothill status at the best of times. My life is spent at a desk. While in my hospital bed I had an anxious dream in which, as usual, the geography made no sense. One moment I was tramping through somewhere like Derbyshire on lanes that seemed familiar. Next, I was running for miles through a strange city. Finally, I edged against the wind towards a narrow gap between stones beyond which a barren landscape extended to the horizon. A dark and fearful

...c place that I was terrified of entering, of testing myself
...inst.

Today, John and I are staring at the turbulent waves of the
Atlantic Ocean from the cliffs of Yesnaby, thinking about the
future, struggling with the uncertainty of where we will be.
It is easier now that John's mother has gone into residential
care, but she still, understandably, wants to see him regularly.

'I don't want to leave, you know that, but she likes me to
take her out in the car, and for lunch, and ... I feel guilty if
I'm away for too long.'

I feel a burden of guilt too, for putting him in a position
where he is torn.

'True north' is 'direct north' towards the pole, not the place
towards which a compass needle points, which is some
distance away, and moves over time. Locating true north is
essential for accurate navigation, both in our travels but also
in finding our way through life. It's the direction of truth.
Perhaps that is why we talk about a 'moral' compass, that
part inside ourselves, which tells us what we know already,
but have chosen to ignore when faced with a moral dilemma.
What is the 'right' thing to do with our lives?

I don't think religious belief is necessary to lead a 'moral'
life. I have a strong sense of 'right' and 'wrong,' but ceased
believing in an all-seeing God decades ago, despite having a
thoroughly religious education. Raised as an Anglican I felt
more affinity with my grandparents' Methodism. Then as a
lonely and depressed medical student, I was seduced into an
evangelical form of Christianity by a young couple, David
and Anna, from an organization called 'Campus Crusade

for Christ', who spent their lives recruiting lost souls in the Pollock Halls of Residence in Edinburgh. They knocked on my door at a time I was very low.

'Come and spend time with us,' they invited. Looking back now it is easy to see how vulnerable a lonely student can be to religious proselytisers. Once, during my time in halls, I saw an ambulance arrive in the night to take someone who was screaming and shouting away to hospital. 'An overseas student under a lot of pressure to do well,' was the rumour going around the next day, 'they tried to harm themselves'.

Under the influence of Campus Crusade, I started going back to church with a couple of friends at Medical School who were, like several in my year, quite vocal practising Christians. When, back at home in the vacation, I told Dad I was going to Midnight Mass at the Anglican Church down the road he responded, 'What the hell are you doing that for?'

'Because I want to.' I replied, but there were tears on my cheek as I walked down the street in the dark. My father's socialism and atheism were inextricable. I always disappointed him.

The evening I told Anna that I intended to move in with my boyfriend, whom I later married, she was horrified. 'It's not the right thing! I do understand, you know, I haven't always been the person I am now, I was lost once, just like you.'

I couldn't imagine that. She seemed very assured of her place in the world and cocooned within a loving family. 'But it feels right for me, now,' I argued.

I never heard from her again.

Since then I've gone through life without the comfort blanket of Christianity, even though at heart I'm still a non-conforming cultural Methodist, with a need to cut through the crap and get to what really matters. That was one of the reasons I never qualified as a psychotherapist. When my supervisor asked me to think about going on a local training course which was rather heavy on Freud, I told him it felt a little like asking me to join a religion. He replied, to my surprise, 'I know what you mean!' I still struggle with any kind of evangelism, but especially on how we manage our mental health.[9] Nevertheless, faith groups can provide companionship and support and a way of making sense of experience.

With warmth and common sense, the Catholic chaplain at the hospital in South Manchester gently counselled a depressed elderly lady who was convinced she had been possessed by the devil and had overdosed on sleeping tablets. 'I told her God still loves her, and will forgive her,' he said to me, 'and to talk to you about the Devil part of it. I told her you can help her with that.' Many people who are bereaved find comfort from talking to a minister, rabbi or imam. Others find it difficult to admit they feel life is not worth living and may believe God has forsaken them.

The most religious place I ever worked was Lancashire, once a stronghold of pre-reformation Catholicism, and the only place where I ever visited a convent to see a nun, a member of a cloistered order, in the confines of her cell. She was very low in mood, seriously physically unwell, and being cared for by older members of the Order. 'She shouldn't be here,' one of them confided. 'This place isn't good for her. She needs to be out in the world.'

Another person I visited in her bedroom, which she rarely left because of unremitting depression, was a Sikh woman who had married a Muslim man.

'How did you meet him?'

'In the street,' she smiled at the memory. 'We fell in love, but our families hated it.' Marriage led to ostracism from both communities and a difficult life at the margins.

Yet, even though I have witnessed both the positives and negatives of religious belief, there is something about seeking a shared sense of spirituality that draws me towards understanding.

Christianity was enforced on the Haida people by missionaries in the nineteenth century. On the sites of their villages, many of the great cypress logs that formed the corner and roof poles of the longhouse now form 'nurseries' for younger spruce that have grown into the canopy since the abandonments of more than a century ago.

'We believe that there are evil spirits in the ground, but they made us bury our dead there.'

You cannot land at a village site without the permission of the Haida *watchman* who lives at the village throughout the summer and receives visitors. Ours was actually a watchwoman, a young mother with her child asleep on her back. She guided us around the village from which her ancestors originally came.

'They made us burn our totem poles for firewood. The ones that remained were taken away by the universities and museums.' There was pain in her voice, but also determination.

'Why did they accept the new ways?' one of the other visitors asked.

'After smallpox killed so many, the missionaries said they could save us. They had nothing else to try.'

First, they brought death. Then, they offered themselves as saviours.

Yet the Haida people did survive and their culture is recovering as they rediscover their old strengths and skills. New totem poles are rising everywhere, telling stories of the families who live in a home or commemorating a life, a history told in elaborately carved eagles, ravens, bears, pine martens and other wild creatures. Hope and renewed meaning are achieved by reconnection with their heritage. Something I can identify with as I rediscover my own.

'The journey did me a great deal of good,' I tell John. He is packing and will be off tomorrow morning on the Hamnavoe.

'I can see that, but I was really worried about you. You know that don't you?' I hadn't been well enough to travel. 'You didn't get permission from your GP. You just went to see her after you came out of hospital and told her you were going, and then things went awry when you got to America.'

'I hadn't realised that you need an electronic visa for Canada now and ...' I called him, in tears, from a New York hotel because I couldn't board until that was sorted out. Neither mind nor body were functioning properly. Even a seasoned traveller makes mistakes but that seriously dented my confidence and gave him more cause for concern.

'I don't think you should be travelling so far on your own.'

'I come up here alone!'

That's different, but I can see this is going nowhere and sigh very loudly.

He puts his arm around my shoulders, 'Look, I was

worried about you. All the time. You know that I don't want you to travel on your own now.'

'You do know I have to be able to. Don't you?'

So many of the uncertainties facing me – of how to live my life – mirror those that I, and my adolescent friends, spent hours talking about fifty years ago. To move forwards I have to do some reconnecting with my past, and that needs to be done alone.

I'm not sure if there is a distinct kind of 'existential' depression, but I have met people whose musings over the apparent pointlessness of life and the inevitability of death contributed to their condition. One of my patients, Andrew, was an exceptionally bright young man who felt trapped in his career and life after university.

'Is there anything that helps you to feel better?' I asked.

'You won't laugh at me if I tell you?'

'No ...' I promise.' Maybe I shouldn't have said that, but I did.

'Football,' he replied.

'Playing it?'

'No. I've worked out that when Rovers are doing well in the league, that's when my mood is up, and when they are on a losing streak, like now, I lose interest in everything ...' He paused for a moment. 'So, I guess there's not much I can do is there?'

Given they were heading for relegation at the time, he was probably right. Life felt beyond his control in every way, and the fortunes of his local football club were the focus, but probably not the only cause, of his misery and despair.

Existential therapists have always explored the concerns

that people have about life's great questions. There are said to be four primary issues that thoughtful people contemplate at various points in their life: that death is an inevitability; we possess freedom but have to create a structure for ourselves within this world; we are fundamentally always isolated because, however close we become to another person, there is always a gap that cannot be bridged; if we must die, what does it all really mean anyway? We brood about these things when we are young and return to think about them if we have therapy or counselling but then work, health and families take over until we have time to think about them again.

After my father died, and I failed my professional examination to become a psychiatrist, my carefully constructed view of myself, and the world with which I had tried so hard to conform, fell apart ... but that was just the beginning. It is hard to go back once you see the pretences and inconsistencies of your life, but falling apart, or 'dis-integrating', can sometimes be a positive thing. With therapy, we try to find a new way forward, to feel whole again, and live by our own rules rather than trying to please others. We check our lives against our own true north at various times in our lives.

It is early September and Orkney's dark autumnal skies are filled with geese in transit, flying in their familiar V formation, which I always imagine is led by a bad-tempered senior with the flaps of his leather hood trailing as he turns to shout 'keep up.' Sitting at my desk, I am writing about the climax of the Canadian expedition.

After two days, we reached our furthest point into the wilderness: the world heritage site of *SGang Gwaay* and a row of totem poles that has stood for over a hundred years, since the inhabitants moved to the modern settlement they live in now. The only audible sound came from the waves as they breached the shore, and a watchman, a celebrated modern Haida artist, who told us the story of each carving.

'The poles of the houses are slowly being absorbed by the forest. Doesn't that make you feel kind of sad?' one of our group asked.

'Everything goes back to the earth eventually,' he said. 'One day each of these poles will fall. It is what is meant to happen.'

We walked back over the crest of the island to the boat, through virgin temperate rainforest of red cedar, spruce and hemlock, drunk with the heavy scent of dark earth and damp, lush vegetation spread with a seamless down of moss. More hung from the trees like tinsel on a Christmas tree and unfamiliar fungi colonised the stumps. Even the light which filtered through the canopy was tinged green. This was exactly as I have always imagined the underworld. It was eerie, not of this world, and I felt disappointed when we emerged into the light because in that other place time seemed to be suspended.

During those few days I began to feel more optimistic than I had since receiving my diagnosis of kidney disease. Having recovered from sepsis, a life-threatening disease, I became more at ease with the future. I have the freedom to make of it what I choose, but the anxiety that has been with me all my life still exists and will probably never leave.

However, there was something about Haida Gwaii that reminded me of the Buddhist concept of the flow of life. Like the forest plants all around them, the remains of the villages will be recycled by nature. This is the reality of our existence.

We make the most of the life we have, however brief, but the outcome is inevitable. What are we going to do with our time? What really matters to us?

There is something about caring for others *in extremis* that touches the core of who we are. It can enhance us through reflection on the profound questions of what it means to be human, but it can, in equal strength, damage us and leave us less capable of responding with humanity.

It is very hard to separate 'me' from the doctor I trained to be. My 'self' has become altered by being entwined both with my professional persona and the lives of my patients, and it is difficult to tell my story without recourse to the clinical tales that illustrate it. Now, the stories filed in my memory are those of people I meet along the way.

Our guide, Mike, was a young Canadian who told us that he had gone to university to study science. 'It wasn't the right thing for me, so I dropped out to work in tourism and conservation,' he told us.

He spent his summers guiding tourists on expeditions like ours and had an immense knowledge of the places he visited. He knew all the Haida watchmen and pointed out to us how the forest might look if it were virgin and untouched. Here and there, if you knew where to look, were the marks that man had left. For example, where bark had been stripped from cedar trees the surrounding bark curled inwards but didn't succeed in obliterating the gap. Cedar bark has many uses, including weaving the traditional hats worn by the Haida people. The marks they made on their world can still be seen generations later. Some of the trees are hundreds of years old.

Mike had taken good care of us all, including me when I fell on the boardwalk between the ruined houses and broke my glasses. At one village, the two resident watchmen, a retired Canadian Mounted Policeman and his wife, greeted us with freshly baked 'fry bread' and cinnamon buns. Mike obviously had a strong relationship with them and there was visibly mutual respect and kindness. One of the other women in our group could not believe that he was the same age as her son and daughter-in-law, both hard working medics.

'Maybe I've not grown up yet,' he laughed. In some ways, perhaps he hadn't.

I couldn't help but tell him, 'Don't grow up.' For a moment I felt like a fool, a psychiatrist saying that to someone I barely knew. But growing up, or at least what 'grown ups' under-stand that to be, is overrated. Our path to adulthood can be traumatic and we can find ourselves following a route that seems to be right and proper but is ultimately unsustainable. Sooner or later we must recover our strength and find another direction. As a therapist, I sought to help patients recognise what they valued. Our values are the principles by which we make judgments about what is important in life. What seems right for us at this point in our lives, not what a doctor or therapist thinks is best.

Like the Haida bark stripper, I always wanted to leave a lasting mark on the world. With a strong need to support the underdog and a powerful belief that being a woman should not prevent me from doing anything, my inability to keep my mouth shut in the face of injustices at work cost me greatly in terms of mental health. I'm moving forward now on a path shared with John and that means negotiation, which I admit I'm not always thoughtful about.

'When are you coming back to Yorkshire?' he asks tonight, as we talk on Skype. It is still light at 10 o'clock and, up the hill, my neighbour is once again taking advantage of the dry late summer weather to cut the hay in his fields. The drones and clanging of farm machinery bounce around the valley.

'A couple of weeks, but I am getting quite a lot of writing done. It's going well.'

'Good for you! I wish I could say the same. I'm looking forward to us having more time together again. I do wish I was back up there with you.' There is a wistfulness in his voice I have heard before. He thinks we have been apart for too long.

On the last day in the wilderness of Gwaii Haanas, we landed at a place called Windy Bay where a huge new totem pole stood in a clearing. There was almost no trace of the original buildings.

'This was raised to commemorate the fight to save this place, and the achievement of winning the battle against the loggers,' the watchwoman told us. She pointed to the cabin nearby. 'This is where the five people who led the resistance lived while this was happening in the eighties, and here,' she pointed to the figures on the pole near about two-thirds the way down, 'you can see them represented. One of the figures has gumboots on. There are some theories about why that is.' She didn't elaborate.

Some of the loggers joined the demonstrations even though to do so would damage their livelihoods, because they came to believe that cropping a paradise on earth was morally wrong. This was the place that thirty years ago the National Geographic reported was about to be mechanically cleared when the people, some very strong women amongst them, stood up for what they believed and joined arms in front of the trucks. They thought it was the right thing to do, and history has supported them. They saved the Gwaii Haanas for us all.

Finding my way back to my own True North means remembering what really mattered to me before work and career took over my life. It is a journey not only of recovery but also re-*dis*covery of what mattered before, and after, that first journey here to Orkney.

John and I need to find a balance between our need to be alone, and to be together, but it isn't easy, and while you only dream about the future you can't be disappointed by it. It is time for us get on and make the most of it.

'I would like to go back to Haida Gwaii someday,' I tell him before we say goodbye. Outside, the blue and red hues of a darkening mackerel sky predict another change in the weather. 'Next time let's travel together. What do you think?'

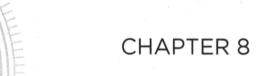

CHAPTER 8

Happy to feel sad

After two months away from Orkney the house is bone-chillingly cold. I returned to Yorkshire in mid-September, and now it is November. The horizontal rain has found its way under the ill-fitting frame of the front door, soaking the junk mail piling up behind it. The bottle of olive oil in the kitchen has solidified into a brick. My island home seems to groan with displeasure at being left alone. Both stoves are stacked with fuel, ready for lighting, but it takes a couple of hours before the heat begins to penetrate. Wrapping myself in a patchwork blanket on the chaise longue, I risk taking off my woolly hat, but my nose is freezing, and the bedroom can only be faced with two hot water bottles. I will myself to sleep in the hope that when I wake the 'Wee Hoose' will forgive my neglect and resume our previously warm relationship.

The last couple of weeks has been particularly eventful. Suddenly and unexpectedly, John's mother died, and he is struggling to come to terms. I am ashamed of my sense of relief, but now we can get on with the rest of our lives, which seem to have been 'on hold' for years.

'What have you been doing today?' I ask him on skype.

'Sorting out stuff . . .' He looks tired. 'I've got to get copies of the death certificate tomorrow. There's a lot to do.'

'I am sorry I had to come away . . .'

'I know,' he interrupts, 'but there isn't much you can do here.' There never is, and I can see how conflicted he is, missing the warm and loving mother she once was.

'I wish I was there to hug you,' or could reach through the screen and embrace him.

'You have things to do. Don't worry about me.'

My heart is aching for John. I want to be with him, to hold him and hug him, but I am conflicted too, feeling better in body and mind than for a long time.

Next day there is a meeting about mental health care on the island, reviewing how local services need to change to address the wellbeing of the people of Orkney. The problem is that we aren't sure what 'well-being' means. It's defied definition for hundreds of years.

Some psychologists define it as 'feeling good and functioning well'. If that is the case, many do not achieve well-being. We are told off for talking about our problems and symptoms rather than 'recognising our strengths'. Governments now regularly measure 'well-being' and the economist Lord Layard, who promotes getting everyone with mental health problems recovered and back to work, has written a book entitled *Happiness*. However, we should be suspicious of economists who measure happiness as they might simply be in search of quick ways to get us back into harness.

Since emerging from my last 'brain fog', and feeling much better after returning from Canada, I've started to register how much people suffer under both the harshness of 'austerity' and the awful uncertainty of overarching politics in the era of populism.

'You get very self-absorbed when you are down,' John has told me.

The nature of depressed mood means that we view everything through bleakly tinted spectacles, and there is a curious narcissism associated with depression. We think too much about ourselves, but as I begin to see the world with sharper focus, I am fairly sure that it is not just about me. It really is looking dank and grey.

In Kirkwall's huge leisure centre, the Pickaquoy Centre (which everyone calls the 'Picky Centre') several people report how difficult it is to access the kind of help they need, difficulties that are exacerbated by cuts to services. There is a tremendous turnout for a small island community, more than sixty people, and we are delighted that so many want to tell those in positions of power what the current difficulties are, including the local Member of the Scottish Parliament. A woman gets up to speak.

'I have a diagnosis of bipolar disorder.' Her voice trembles for a moment before she gets into her stride. 'I know when my mood is going down, but I just can't get an appointment, and I know it will get worse if I don't get help soon.'

Another person, a man this time, tells us, 'I needed someone to talk to, but my doc told me that he couldn't get me seen by the service. There are people here who have helped me, and I want to thank them, but it really needs to be better than this.'

'We *can* do better than this,' someone else says, taking up the theme to a general murmur of agreement.

Yes, we can, but to do that we have to recognise that

everyone needs help tailored to their individual needs. No two of us suffer in quite the same way. What happens to me may or may not echo with another person's experience, although some of it probably will. Some question whether 'depression' even exists; is it simply a form of unhappiness? By calling it 'depression' are we medicalising misery and turning normal sadness into illness? Whatever we call it, severely depressed people suffer differently and need something that takes those differences into account.

After the meeting closes, I walk into the darkness to unwind, and to find a stronger cup of coffee. The Christmas decorations are already lit and the inviting shop windows full of gifts, though it isn't yet December. In the middle of Kirkwall's main street is the Big Tree, a two-hundred-year-old sycamore. I remember it clearly from forty years ago, because everyone told me there are no trees in Orkney, and here was one right in town. Actually there are plenty if you know where to look, but this is the most famous. Spindly, supported by a concrete post, perhaps a little tired of life, but still standing.

An old colleague, a former mental health nurse who teaches meditation down in Yorkshire and lived in Orkney for a couple of years in his youth, told me once how a letter addressed simply to 'Don, near the Big Tree, Kirkwall', reached him at his flat above the shops. He also lived for a while in the Khyber Pass. Not on the Pakistan-Afghanistan Border but a dark passage between old houses in Stromness. The store where I settle down for a more powerful brew is a colourful emporium of knitwear, gifts and food, but there is a sense of sadness in the air, as another year comes towards an end. For me, it isn't an unwelcome feeling at all.

So many people seem to be in pursuit of *happiness* by spending money on 'unique' experiences, refashioning their lives by reading books or going for therapy. If they don't achieve happiness the conclusion will not be anything to do with life's difficulties such as the traumas of childhood, the struggles of poverty, or the lack of meaningful employment. The kind of stories told in the Picky Centre are about the real difficulties that people have. In this age of relentless positivity, the conclusion may be that you simply haven't been trying, or smiling, hard enough to change.

I tell John about the meeting this evening. 'There was a cartoonist drawing at the back. I managed to offend him though, so I'm not sure how he will portray me ...'

'What did you do?'

'Put my coffee down on his table ... I didn't realise what he was doing.'

'You have a history with coffee cups ...'

'I do tend to leave them everywhere.'

How have we lived together 'happily' for so long, when we are so very different? I am tidier than I used to be, he is perhaps a little less of a curmudgeon when it comes to having everything in its place. We have slowly accommodated, but it is tricky for both of us. We are far from happy with each other all the time.

'I hope I can see the finished drawing,' I tell him.

There is a view that the 'positive psychology' movement has pervaded almost every aspect of the twenty-first century through its influence on business, economic theories and health care. We have been fooled into believing that if we want something enough it will happen, that if we can only be optimistic about recovering from cancer, we will. Sadly, there is little or no evidence for this. Reading daily 'affirmations' and writing gratitude letters about what is good in their lives isn't going to improve things for the people of Orkney who have difficulty with everyday living. They need people who will listen and can provide help.

This summer, in my favourite bookshop, the Elliott Bay Book Company on the top of Capitol Hill in Seattle, on the way back from Canada, I discovered that the 'personal development' shelves have been relabelled as 'self'. On the top of this section was now a sign that simply said 'self-overstock' which might or might not be ironic. I didn't purchase anything, though I did buy a large vanilla cone from the ice-cream shop next door, which provided relatively short-lived but exquisite pleasure.

What really made me happy was seeing my friend Loryn again after almost a year. She hugged me when we met. 'Are you sure you should be travelling again so soon? How is John?'

Happiness has as much, if not more, to do with how we interact with others than what we do ourselves. We need to find the right balance between the stresses and support we experience from being with them. That's the hard part, and it is something that John and I have spent decades working on.

Sitting in the living room, which is no longer warmed by the greenhouse effect of the two skylights as it was in summer, I meditate by breathing in and out while focusing on the sensation of air travelling through my trachea, throat, pharynx and nostrils. Imagining myself as someone wise and compassionate, I try to feel like I am that person, or more crucially, that a part of me is. After trying to be such a person for patients, friends and my husband over so many years, is it possible that I can be such a person for me?

Many of my books are in Orkney now. Arranged on shelves beside the living-room fireplace, the collection is supplemented by purchases from the local bookshop in Stromness. It looks as if it hasn't changed much in the last half century and advertises itself as a 'drive through'. There is no pavement in much of the main street, the cobbled highway is shared by people, cars, and the local feline population including one large ginger affectionately nicknamed 'Speed-bump'. The shop is a great place to burrow through every now and then for things to challenge my brain and is highly celebrated. There is a painting of it, and its owner, in the library. I thought I had stopped buying self-help books after taking so many to the charity bookshop in Yorkshire, but some have managed to find their way into the boxes I brought here.

The only one I've continued to read these last few months has been Paul Gilbert's book *The Compassionate Mind*. I want to carry on learning about meditation even though my experience with mindfulness in the spring wasn't particularly positive. What is so good about Gilbert's writing is that he doesn't promise everything, nor suggest that it is all down to you. That if you don't work hard enough you have only yourself to blame if you don't feel better. It's a kind and gentle approach, a kind of 'try out some of these ideas as you might find them helpful'. He talks about allowing yourself a 'slight, gentle smile' as you think about what it is like to be compassionate and forgiving.

I've been trying it out, and those familiar sensations in my chest that I associate with loss flood into consciousness. Yet there is something different today. Instead of feeling afraid of being overwhelmed by pangs of sadness, I can tolerate those sensations and even welcome them. I can raise a gentle, even wry, smile at the idea that all the things I expect of myself could be possible. Imagining myself in this white painted room surrounded by my precious objects: the Egyptian cat god Bast on the mantelpiece, the exquisite porcelain lion I bought from a potter this summer, an old photograph of our cat Sophie. Being here on this tiny speck of an island at almost 59 degrees north, for less than a hundred thousand millionth of a gnat's breath (still a gross overestimate) of duration in the stream of life and time, doesn't engender a sense of calm exactly, but I feel different. Much more in touch with the world than earlier in the year.

'Do what makes you anxious, not what makes you depressed,' I was told by my friend who meditates. In other words: recognise the difference between acceptance of something difficult, and simply being resigned to it and at its mercy. I'm still not sure I can get my head around that. Acceptance isn't easy if you are an angry person for whom the injustices of life trigger incandescent rage. Perhaps I am wilfully misunderstanding the concept.

'I've been sorting out some of the stuff that was left in the house when Mum moved into the care home,' John tells me.

It is always challenging, going through the remnants of a family life. The emotions, that a box full of forgotten belongings can provoke, defy the simple solutions offered by 'three easy steps' those 'decluttering' books promise.

'How are you?'

'I'm OK. I just keep finding photographs, and postcards, and old toys. It's a journey into the past and ... it leaves you ...' his voice falters.

'A bit wrung out ...'

There are things from his childhood that he intends to bring back from his parents' old home. He wants to show them to me. Especially the little bear with its fur worn thin in the shape of a tiny hand. His mother kept it as a special memento and embarrassed him early in our relationship by showing it to me. 'Enjoy being in Orkney, I know you always do,' he signs off, 'but don't forget that I miss you, and I wish you were here.'

Then he is gone, and I am alone again.

For some of us, relationships with family can be so fractured that we never gather together such things to remember them by, and never want to. For others, those trinkets bequeathed to us can cause considerable pain.

Once I spent several consultations with a patient just trying to help us both make some sense of the complex web of relationships between adults and children that comprised her 'family tree', a tangle of infidelity, abuse, violence and abandonment, on a large sheet of paper. Those meetings helped us to understand where the problems in her life arose and begin to understand why certain things her mother had left to her, particularly her wedding ring, distressed her so much.

All that remains from my childhood are a few photographs and books and pieces of jewellery: a watch and silver bracelet given to me by my father. The memories that haunt me are more often triggered by place.

At the end of the summer I visited New Lanark on the way

to Yorkshire, having never visited before. The road spiralled through the Clyde valley until it finally arrived at the top of a hill looking down on streets of terraced cottages clinging to the slopes and a row of giant mills curving around the river-bank, with one huge chimney. All around this harsh urban architecture, greenery and dense woodland covered the hills.

Sometimes it feels like we are back in a time of Dickensian values, but the ideals on which New Lanark was founded are far from the traditions of the workhouse. A sign attached to the iron railings by one of the doorways reads:

> '*In this new world all will know that far more happiness can be obtained by union, than by disunion.*'

It's a quotation from the person who helped to establish New Lanark, the visionary Victorian entrepreneur and philanthropist Robert Owen, who by strange coincidence, so I read today, began as a textile manufacturer in Manchester, and later in Chorlton-on-Medlock, close to where I started work as a psychiatrist.[10] Owen was right. Happiness is more likely achieved with others than by focusing on ourselves, but early relationships may get in the way rather than prepare us for it.

My roots are near New Lanark, yet so far away too. Until recently I drove up through this part of Scotland, where half of my genes originated, without visiting my mother's place of birth. Out of touch with my heritage I had cut out another part of my life. My maternal grandfather was a miner in the Lanarkshire coalfield, and my uncle a steelworker at Ravenscraig near Motherwell, both now long gone. On holidays, I shared a bed with two of my cousins in the Whitehill council estate, one of the first places in Britain to impose a youth curfew. It wasn't pretty, and I was always aware that I didn't fit in. I didn't speak with the same accent, didn't have (quite) the same approach to alcohol and wasn't preoccupied with blue or green on a Saturday afternoon. I had absolutely no idea who the Catholics were in my class at school, but at least we all went to the same one.

So, I was bemused when my cousin felt the need to inform an eight-year-old me, as we stood outside in the street, 'See that family up there in that house? They're Catholics . . . and so are they.' He pointed in the opposite direction.

Later, I became aware that my grandfather, whom I never knew, had belonged to the local Orange Lodge and was active in the sectarian tradition of central Scotland. When my relationship with my mother deteriorated to the point that we cut off contact, it became harder to feel affinity with the place of her birth. My mother's family, rather like her, were mystified by my desire to get an education. They couldn't wait to get out to work and earn a living. To me their world seemed small. To them, on my visits from Edinburgh, I was somewhere between a snob and a dreamer.

So, as I wandered around the mills of New Lanark and looked over the fast-flowing Clyde it wasn't my mother this place called to mind, but my father. The values of its founder reminded me of him and his anger at the inequalities of life. As memories rushed back, I felt unutterably sad . . . and yet it didn't overwhelm me. I was almost happy to experience the quality of sadness at what might have been. If only he hadn't died so young. If only we had mended fences before he died, and a hundred other versions of 'if only'.

*

Sadness is not depression. It is a normal human emotion but a powerful one that provides us with a message. It signals thoughts and feelings we need to work on, process and resolve. Resisting the experience of sadness can, paradoxically, lead to a welling up of such intense darkness that we become numb and stop feeling altogether. Recovery from depression means being able to feel the complete range of human emotions. It is not about being 'happy' although we may experience periods of happiness and pure joy along with sadness, anger, hope, fear and the whole gamut of moods and emotions.

Moments of acute sadness can rise during mindfulness practice and may be hard to deal with. Some sadness can be productive and can open us to a sense of being connected, in the same flow of life. However, to imagine ourselves in the presence of a compassionate other who cares about us can be rather scary. What if they disappoint us, leave us or let us down? We hold ourselves aloof, politely dismissive of the kind words of others, afraid to acknowledge our own neediness.

The feeling for me is that if I should give in to my thirst for kindness it would never be slaked. My soul would soak it up like blotting paper with a bottle of spilt ink. The compassion I felt for others in my work wasn't experienced as 'happiness' but as a painful awareness of the empathic connection I had with those who were still suffering.

As I once learned how to be with people in pain, so I am learning how to be with myself.

As the evening chill sets in, I light the kitchen fire and start to prepare a meal, shedding a few tears as I chop an onion.

Slicing garlic, browning the chicken and frying spices for a curry – ginger, cardamom, cumin and turmeric – until their heady scent rises above the pan, I realise I'm taking pleasure from cooking for the first time in years. At the back of the kitchen table, against the wall where the radio connects me with the world beyond, is the dish in which I keep the tablets that I still take every day. Fewer antidepressants now, but I am back again on the pills for my blood pressure. The effect of the sepsis wasn't long lasting. No-one disturbs me here, and there is plenty of time to think. The cows are back in their barn, their voices carrying on the evening breeze from the farm where Katie the cat lived. Beneath the ridge of hills over which Hoy can be seen in daylight is a place known locally as 'Happy Valley'. If it were still light it would just be possible to see the tops of the trees from my garden. Many different species, sycamore, beech, oak, elm, apples, rowan and even a Monkey Puzzle tree were planted decades ago by a local farmer who wanted to create his own place of beauty. It's extraordinary how they have thrived in Orkney. In the spring, bluebells carpet the woodland. There are no signs to it from the main road, and now although mostly bare and barren it will still be beautiful in its stark winter garb.

Generally, when people recover from severe depression, they don't expect to feel happy. They just want to be 'normal' again, to be able to feel *something*, because when you are very low you don't feel very much at all.

When you are severely depressed it is almost impossible to be creative in any way. Yet the melancholic state which inspired Keats to pen *Ode to Autumn* and the reclusive Emily Dickinson to create a collection of poems virtually unread in her lifetime clearly wasn't mental paralysis. Creative melancholy exists as a contemplation of the world tinged with a sometimes bleak yet ultimately realistic state of sadness. Being able to access our normative experience of sadness, without the constant fear that we will spiral into the depths of depression, allows us to ponder complicated thoughts about the present constructively. When we see problems through a realistic lens, we begin to resolve them. It is a place where many people create their most complex and meaningful art.

There is something too about the idea of being in the North that evokes for me a kind of romantic melancholy, a yearning for solace in the darkness of winter. I know that bittersweet feeling well. There is a poignant sadness when I think about Katie. It wasn't the right time for me to have another feline companion, but the intense pain of losing Sophie, and the depression it triggered, are long gone. I am happy to be able to feel sad. Because, as the values of New Lanark and the work I've done in Orkney remind me, there is still much to do for those who find themselves at the mercy of injustice.

This evening, I tell John what I have been writing about, as I often do. He is understandably very sad, for he is grieving. 'Are you sure that you are OK?' he asks me.

'Yes, I am good. I've been writing today . . . trying to make sense of what to expect when we recover from depression.'

'And . . . '

'Well, it isn't so much happiness as the ability to experience intense moments.'

Talking to him reminds me how human beings make a habit of capturing those flashes of happiness in photographs. The picture on my computer screen was taken by John in

Edinburgh during my recovery from sepsis, when slouched in a chair in our room in the Caledonian Hotel. I'd been awarded the Presidential Medal by the Royal College of Psychiatrists. All year, since receiving the letter, I'd not really believed it. It didn't fit with the script in which I was an imposter who had not achieved much in life.

'You look relaxed and happy,' John told me when he showed it to me.

Reliving that moment now, months after the event, sitting in my woven chair in a semi-dark room lit only by the lamp at my desk and the glow of the evening fire from the stove next to me, I share a confiding smile with my reflection on the other side of the window glass, in the silent night.

CHAPTER 9

Meaning and Hope

It is almost Christmas and an icy wind is blowing through Kirkwall. Despite being swathed in multiple layers of wool I am still freezing but enjoying bright, cold days. The street is busy with people doing their last-minute shopping. We've been searching for the right sized dish in which to cook our first Christmas roast in Orkney.

'What are you thinking about?' I ask John.

He pauses before replying. 'I was wondering if you wanted to have some cake.'

I look over at the sideboard, covered in mouth-watering pastries. I am slouching with my elbows on the table as I always do, looking directly at him now with my chin supported by my interlocked fingers. 'Silly question.'

Someone opens the door behind us, and the wind whistles in. 'Actually,' he exhales and his shoulders sag a little, 'I was thinking that this is the first Christmas I've not had to think about Mum ... what's happening to her, how will we ferry her around for dinner at our place ... that sounds awful doesn't it?'

I reach out and squeeze his hand. 'No, it doesn't . . . maybe it's time for you to live your life again.'

It's a time when cheerfulness seems mandatory, but it's hard for those without families or support. I always rehearsed with my patients how they were going to cope alone. After separation from my first husband, and alienation from family, I spent a few Christmases alone. Fortunate that I could afford to travel, I escaped to France, walking the streets of Paris and the boardwalk at Deauville, learning how to experience and enjoy my own company once more. Times that are memorable not only because of the novelty of rebuilding a life by revisiting places alone, but also the generosity of others. Discovering that the tyre on my mini was flat on Christmas Eve, and incapable of changing it, I arrived at a garage in Normandy where the mechanics were about to go home. Reluctant at first to help, one of them asked where I was from.

'I've driven all the way from Manchester.'

'Manchester?' he paused, '*Manchester United*?'

'Yes, yes!' I replied, though at work I always tried to remain neutral on the football question. Springing into action, he had my car back on the road in minutes.

'I'm really very well at the moment and feeling better physically than I have for years,' I told my psychiatrist a week ago when I saw him in Manchester.

He looked up from writing in my notes. 'Oh, that's good!'

'Following the advice I used to give to patients, about how sleep affects mood, I've been going to bed earlier.'

'It really works . . . ' he put down his pen, 'You seem as well as I have known you this last few years.' We shared that knowing smile that only doctors exchange about how we unfailingly expect others to 'do as I say but not as I do'.

'Is there any news yet about whether the Mood Disorders service will carry on?' I knew there had been a stay of execution, but the decision was still up for review.

'Nothing yet, but it's not looking likely.'

'Oh . . . ' It was difficult to hide my disappointment. 'Something else has happened . . . ' I couldn't remember how much I had told him about this. 'For years I had symptoms of an infection. Ever since they diagnosed the kidney disease. They could never find anything but now, since the antibiotics in hospital, they've completely gone.'

'Really?'

'My GP thinks I might have had a chronic infection all this time.' Not wanting him to enjoy the irony of an expert in medically unexplained symptoms experiencing them herself, I had kept silent.

'Ah,' he smiled, 'You know we are beginning to understand how chronic inflammation in any part of the body can make depression worse for people who have severe mood problems.'

Although inflammation is the latest biological explanation for depression, part of me has always been sceptical about the simplicity of biomedical theories. Yet something has changed in me. Is it bacterial, emotional or both, and might I have a second chance at life? A patient with 'medically unexplained symptoms', back at the beginning of my career, had been similarly convinced that she had an infection.

Hilda had visited the emergency department at the hospital several times every month, and seen numerous consultants, but no-one could explain her symptoms, other than they must be 'psychological' or 'supratentorial'[11] as some doctors used to write in their letters. It wasn't a compliment.

'I'm not mad! You don't think I'm mad do you, Doctor?' she remonstrated.

'No, I don't think you are, but you are very, very upset by these symptoms.'

'You think they are real? You believe me? Nobody ever listens.'

'I do, but I don't think it's possible to make them go away,' I said. 'I can see how unhappy you are ... '

'You don't believe me! No-one does.'

Hilda found it impossible to 'learn to live the best quality life you can despite the symptoms' as everyone, including me, kept telling her. I feel ashamed that we didn't take her seriously enough and, knowing how my persistent symptoms were treated, recall her now with growing empathy. Her doctors, including me, just wanted her to resign herself, so she gradually lost hope. With experience, I learned to carry the torch of hope for my patients. When they didn't see how things could be better, they believed I did.

However, when we get past the stage of just surviving, we need more than hope. We have to prevent the darkness returning and start to ask ourselves questions like: 'What am I going to do with the rest of my life?' 'What does all this really mean?' and most difficult of all, 'Is this all there is going to be?'

It isn't a white Christmas, just windy. Not unusual for Orkney. The willow branches that in summer were beginning to obscure the view from my desk are bare, stark and tremulous in the breeze. It's the kind of day when it isn't safe to go outside with a large piece of cardboard for fear of ending up in the next field. There is no wind quite like the wind of Orkney. The air is almost always in motion. A short walk against the wind can feel so invigorating that you think you have taken far more exercise than you have, using both more energy to push harder and having your bronchial tubes spring-cleaned. Then on the way back its easier as you are wind-assisted.

When I bought this house, it came with a wooden shed which, like so many light structures in north and west Scotland, had been chained to the ground. 'A few days after it was built it flew into our field,' Mary, my neighbour told me a while ago. When the shed door blew shut I couldn't get out because the bolt was too rusted. I had to kick it open or I might have been in there until the postman tried to leave a parcel.

Unable to move after eating our Christmas pudding, we settle into the cosy warmth of the living room, in front of the stove, and by early evening, not long after the watery sun has disappeared over the horizon, John falls sound asleep. He is exhausted.

On the chaise longue, trying to concentrate on my book, my thoughts wander into the future. The new shed in my garden, with its solid white walls, is the first building I have ever had constructed from scratch. Is this a sign that I am ready to put down roots? If so, is John too? Is this still what he wants?

Shining directly into my eyes, today's sun is sinking towards the horizon behind Hoy, even though it is barely mid-afternoon. It made an unexpected appearance half an hour ago which prompted John to get his camera equipment together.

'That's the advantage of winter here, you don't have to

get up early for sunrise – or stay up late for sunset,' he says.

Photography has always been his passion. Perhaps second only to cats, but now we are cat-free it has moved to top spot. It isn't that he wants to exhibit his pictures. I struggle to get him to show them at all. He wants to take photographs that he is satisfied with, to master the skills. Unlike me, he doesn't feel an urgent drive to achieve perfection in whatever he does.

At my desk with the blind drawn halfway down now, the glass of water on the shelf behind my laptop screen refracts the sharp winter sunlight. It reminds me of a painting that John and I bought from an artist in the Western Isles years ago – of nothing but light and a glass of water. Simple, yet beautifully executed.

I am writing about a recent journey to the Middle East. Remembering an afternoon of tranquillity when I had been enjoying a warm breeze and reading a book on my hotel balcony. I had come to speak at a conference. These days I don't only experience the interplay of mood and chronic illness, I train others in how to broach the topic of emotions with people who feel stigmatised for being physically ill.

As a friend of mine with physical and mental health challenges has said to me more than once: 'We aren't supposed to feel anxious about our physical health problems, but we do.'

There was something surreal in reading about a writer's experiences in a concentration camp in Poland in 1944 while staring over the cerulean blue waters of the Arabian Gulf, but that was what I was doing. Over the water was the opulent shopping mall I had visited the day before, its glass frontage dazzling in the sunshine, where I had spooned liquid chocolate out of a Martini glass, idly watching as workmen put up Christmas decorations, wondering about how much this fleeting indulgence was going to cost, musing on whether anyone could afford to buy from the deserted luxury shops nearby. Eating alone has never bothered me because I can easily lose myself in the world of a book, my portable bolthole.

Once, at a restaurant in the Tivoli Gardens in Copenhagen, I was so absorbed that I accidentally pushed my table napkin into a candle with the edge of my novel. The paper caught fire and I managed to beat out the flames with the only thing to hand, the paperback! Everyone in the room turned to look as blackened flakes of paper floated over the carpet. Generally, I try hard not to draw attention to myself: the quiet reader seated, like most lone travellers, somewhere by the kitchen door. This was a rare exception.

Dressed as modestly as possible, but with my head uncovered, I tried to remain anonymous in this Middle Eastern city too, but, being European, that wasn't easy. There are few places in the world that seem more alien to me, where the primary value seems to be making money and spending it on the tallest building, or the hotel with the most gravity defying walls. Apart from my taxi driver and the hotel staff, none of whom were natives of the Gulf, I didn't meet any people who had seen this place grow from seaside villages and desert to an international city built on oil. The only moment that touched something inside me was when we drove past two battered Land Rovers parked under makeshift shelters in an old palace courtyard. Our guide told us they had been amongst the late Sheikh's most treasured possessions – and they did not glitter.

My most memorable journeys have been to the homes of people who live and work in a place, not to grand houses and palaces, however exquisite. The apartment in Timişoara in Romania in 1992, not long after the fall of the *Ceauşescu* regime, where I had been wrapped in blankets because the gas supply was cut off. The professor of psychiatry insisted that I ate the wonderful food her mother had brought in from the farm, although there was enough on the table to feed the family for a week and that they might need. Her husband was at home, but I never met him.

'He doesn't feel good now he has no work.' The former research scientist was too depressed, I suspected, to join us.

A few years later, after numerous joyous toasts in a similar apartment in Tomsk, Siberia, my host announced, 'Linda, we are so honoured, so pleased that you have come to visit our home in Russia,' as he lifted his vodka glass once more. I had lost count by then and toasted my journey to another place far in the North. However grim the outside of the soviet apartment blocks, these families had created a home, a place where they belonged, and which gave their life meaning.

Victor Frankl, the psychiatrist who survived Auschwitz, wrote more clearly than anyone else about the human search for meaning. When I read him again, as I did while in the Gulf, I'm struck that the first of the things he mentions is work, something that people with mental health problems are repeatedly told is 'good' for them. Many would consider that dreary work adds to the meaninglessness of existence, but of course it depends how work is defined. It isn't only about earning money. Perhaps everyone has something they feel driven to do, as some of us need to write, but there are the things we must do to satisfy the society we live in, our own conscience and to simply take care of ourselves.

When working with an organisation that encouraged

people with mental illness to rediscover their creativity, I watched how the work of making something with your own hands could aid a person's recovery.

Jane, in her sixties, had felt depressed for many years following the early death of her husband. Looking forward to getting back to her ceramics group each morning, although this was the first time she had tried it, she told me, 'I'm not doing something sad and depressing now, talking about how I'm feeling. This is fun. It's something beautiful.' For her, creating an object was an emotional labour of love, but she had other work to do. 'I have to sort out all the prescriptions for my diabetes and blood pressure . . . get to the appointments with the hospital for my eyes, my feet, my heart.'

The everyday grind of caring for yourself gets harder when you are sick. That too is a form of work.

At first, when suffering severe depression more than twenty years ago, I had been unable to do anything much. Spending all day staring into space I struggled to watch television in the evening. However, as my mood improved, I began, with support from John to reengage with life, covering canvasses and furniture with bright colours and beginning the kind of life I would like to live now.

Sadly, there are tubes of paint in my study in Yorkshire that have hardened with age, waiting for me to unscrew them again. Something in my soul solidified over those barren decades, but I would still tell my patients who were in a hurry to return to work: 'You aren't really well until you are so busy living that you wonder how you will ever fit it in.'

When we can no longer do the things that are damaging our health, we have to find other ways of working.

A few weeks ago, I was with a group of mental health workers, discussing how they might change the way *they* work. 'How can we try and help someone who is struggling to recover, to move forwards in their own way?'

'Asking what they would like to change about their life?' one replied.

'What they want might be impossible anyway,' said another. 'We are under so much time pressure, it's about getting people in and out as quickly as possible, there's no time for long conversations so we give advice.'

'OK, I understand that. But if a person really doesn't feel able to do what you suggest, or they think it's a waste of time, it won't happen. What else could you say? Maybe ... How would you like your life to be different? What's the first very small step you could take?'

It's time for me to take that step.

John isn't convinced that I should carry on with anything to do with mental health care. 'Why do you have to keep going back? You've done that, you've exhausted yourself, it's time for something different in life.'

'I don't know what else to do that I am good at.'

'Why do you always have to be good at it?'

I played the piano as a child, but it is hard to disentangle practice from working for examinations, when anxiety overwhelmed me. I haven't opened the lid for years. My fingers are stiff in the morning now and I sense arthritis just over the horizon. 'When we move from here, I will have to find a good home for the piano,' I told John recently, in Yorkshire. 'Maybe a school.'

'You don't want to take it with you?'

'No, but someone will want it, I'm sure. They will only have to come and take it away.'

My piano playing never flowed effortlessly, but I confess I never practised hard enough. It was never really my own passion but my father's. He had wanted me to take piano lessons because he didn't take the opportunities he had in his own childhood. 'Play *Ain't Misbehavin*, again will you,' he would say, but I would never, in ten lifetimes, perform it with the effortless *joie de vivre* of his hero, Fats Waller.

Ancient Chinese philosophers described something called *Wu-Wei* or 'no trying', a harmonious state which feels like doing nothing while you are performing at the height of brilliance. Everyone will know how paradoxically hard we strive to achieve that sense of effortless living. To stop overthinking the world, put our conscious mind on hold, and just be. Confucians believe that if you try hard to focus on living the right kind of life, to act the part, it will eventually come naturally. However, going down that road risks becoming a slave to the all too familiar downsides of perfectionism: self-criticism, anxiety and depression. Like so many children across the generations, I rebelled because playing the piano wasn't a goal that had meaning for me.

We have to discover our own passions, like John has re-discovered his photography.

However, there is also a large collection of vinyl records and compact discs that I have barely listened to in years. When did I allow music to leave my life? For a short while in my thirties when I sang, accompanied by a friend on piano, I fantasised a life as a jazz singer instead of academia. As a student, I sang with a choir and found it exhilarating, yet I never returned to it, even though it might have helped me feel better. Listening to music allows us to open the door to that state of creative melancholy from which poignant memories emerge.

A couple of years ago I was at a concert during the St Magnus Festival and heard an old Scottish folk song I hadn't sung since my childhood. Suddenly I was transported into the past. It was *Charlie is my Darling* sung by Eddie Reader in concert with the Scottish National Jazz Orchestra. She performed it with the racier lyrics, written by Robert Burns, rather than the version I remembered, but it was the melody that impacted on me. I hadn't thought about it in years, though I could remember singing it at school, and with my mother. We often sang at home, probably the only times she and I were ever in harmony. I can hold a tune regardless of what cacophony is going on, a metaphor perhaps for retaining my sanity.

Sometimes a change of place can enable us to discover new ways to spend our lives and provide us with a sense of renewed meaning. The year living in Seattle let me find out what I was passionate about and allow that hinterland of interests and pleasures to flourish again. I went to galleries and festivals, trying to rediscover my creativity.

On a weekend course found in Bohemian Seattle's *The Stranger* magazine, based on Julia Cameron's inspirational *The Artist's Way*, a group of strangers holed up in a large log cabin with a hot tub in the Cascade Mountains. Our leader had once been a yoga teacher but was now a self-appointed guru in 'reconnecting with your own creative energy'. We cooked together, practised yoga each morning and, in the evening, everyone but me sat in the hot tub drinking wine. Being British I hadn't realised I needed to bring a swimsuit to the mountains in the middle of winter, which didn't stop me liberally quaffing the wine.

I began going to yoga regularly, and to my very first book festival where I listened to a writer talk about her memoir. She inspired me so much that in the following decade I travelled to attend courses with her and began to write regularly. It wasn't so much the inspirational guru but the essence of the place that had liberated me.

Many of us battle with the problem of not trying too hard at life to regain the spontaneity (and, we hope, the joy) of living in the moment. Practising meditation every day when I feel able, but not when my mood is low, is one way of achieving that. I am going to draw and paint again, to rediscover that curious passion for colour. I'll go for long walks, get out of my mind and into my body, and make just enough effort to enjoy and experiment with new experiences, without looking for courses to take and exams to pass or refuse to continue because I do not achieve perfection immediately.

It's getting dark and John hasn't come back. I've tried ringing his mobile phone a couple of times, but it's going to voicemail. Walking up to the lane, I look for headlights coming over the rise. The sky is still lit in silvery blue, as though from behind a silken screen, the blue hour after sunset, but blue-black clouds move across as the light fades back. Down by the main road the streetlights are visible in the gloom. Shivering, I retreat to the kitchen. Ten minutes pass. The front door opens and he comes in, bringing with him the scents of outside: wet wool, clean rain and earth. I get up to hug him and feel how cold and damp he is, his clothes, hands and face.

'How did you get on? I ask. 'It's really late.'

'Not very well. The sun disappeared into a band of cloud. I didn't realise how far I'd walked from the car. It was too windy and wet for the tripod, but I enjoyed getting some air.'

'I was worried. It was getting dark and you might have been blown off the cliffs.' I don't say it, but I'm thinking about what he has told me in the past: times when he felt like ending his life.

We share an ability to embrace the most pessimistic explanation for almost everything that goes wrong in life. We also sometimes imbibe too much alcohol when we are together, the easiest way to achieve that effortless feeling, and the traditional Scots way of getting out of your head. Such a shame it is so bad for us!

Most of the time now, alcohol and I remain on reasonably good terms, but when my mood is low, or I'm under stress, booze still likes to get one up on me. Working full-time, I began to rely a little too much on it, just to avoid thinking. Days were measured on a new scale of severity: the number of bottles of Stella Artois I needed to feel relaxed after a weekday plus the number of glasses of wine and Martinis at the weekend. Mostly I drank just about up to the safe limit for a woman. Sometimes, and increasingly so as time went by, I exceeded it. Alcohol enables me to retreat into that part of me that doesn't care what other people think, the dramatic, passionate woman I can be, but that my other, more disciplined, self cannot tolerate.

While sitting on my balcony in the Gulf as the sun went down over a silver-blue sea, reading about someone trying to stay alive in desperate circumstances, I heard raucous laughter and shouting carried on the breeze from the fake English pub in the garden below. A group of expatriates were getting intoxicated behind hotel walls while paying no attention to a scantily dressed woman who was cheerfully murdering *Yesterday*. It was a curious place to pass the time when life was on pause, and disturbingly without any sense of meaning or authenticity. Alcohol was the perfect antidote to the sensation of dislocation for those marooned here, but I was completely sober and wanted to go home. It was not my idea of paradise.

Optimism is confidence that everything will be fine, but to have hope you must be able to see the road forward. According to Viktor Frankl, who survived not only Theresienstadt, but also Auschwitz, Kaufering and Türkheim, where thousands of Jews were murdered, we can still find meaning in life when confronted with a hopeless situation. People do find meaning in suffering, such as those incredible individuals who turn personal tragedy into triumph by raising money for better research into the cancer that is slowly killing them. Frankl famously said we cannot control what happens to us in life, but we can control how we feel and what we do about it. That is how and why he survived, but we don't all start at the same place, and many cannot do it without the support and compassion of others. Some are too ambivalent to do anything at all and get stuck.

I learned much from a patient, Sue, with lifelong anorexia nervosa. 'People think I hate food,' she told me,' but they don't understand. I think about it all the time. I adore it! I love cooking for others. Food is so important to me, don't you see? Avoiding it helps me to feel in control of my life ... and I feel better, but then ... '

'But then ... ?'

'It's taking over. It's in control of me, and the effect it's having on my life, and my health, is awful. I don't know where to turn.'

It isn't about indecision. It isn't about having no goals for what you want to achieve, but about having conflicting aims. Wanting to have something at the same time as not having it. Wanting to never again experience the pain of loss but craving the end of your loneliness, and so avoiding new relationships. Wanting to both be still here among the living and yet dead and away from it all at the same time. We want the best for ourselves, so we are reluctant to give up any option. It can be disastrous.

The worst thing you can do to someone who is ambivalent is to insist on telling them what to do and how easy that will be for them. It must have really annoyed my father, who smoked forty cigarettes a day, when, as an arrogant medical student, I insisted on telling him why he should stop the habit that would eventually kill him. 'I've seen the evidence, there's a high risk that you will get lung cancer, or heart disease, or emphysema.'

'Don't start telling me what to do – coming back from university with all your ideas. What do you know about life?' Sometimes he would smile while saying this. Other times I could sense his sadness, and anger. 'It's my only pleasure in life. I don't drink, I bring my wage packet home every Friday night and hand it to your mother. I take plenty of exercise. I'm fit for my age.' He walked, cycled and swam until his early death at 52 from coronary artery disease. He never gave up cigarettes, though he knew they were killing him. Listening to himself telling me why there was no point in giving up may have convinced him even more that he was doing the right thing.

It's not comfortable acknowledging your own ambivalence and the choices you fail to take. The fence becomes increasingly narrow and uncomfortable and you have to jump in one direction or the other. You do have the freedom to decide, but if you need help there should be someone there to support you, who understands how difficult it is.

When I look now at the watch he gave to me, saved for with the gift coupons that came with his cigarettes, always hurts. 'Russian,' he said, 'It will last.' Sadly, it stopped working at about the same time as the Soviet Union, outliving him only by a few years. No-one offered him any help to stop then. It was all down to willpower, while the tobacco companies incentivised you to smoke even more.

'We've managed to cut down on alcohol at least,' John says.

It's something my psychiatrist asks about every time that he sees me. Mood and alcohol are intimately entwined. 'When I'm on my own here, I hardly drink at all.'

'So, I lead you astray?'

'You always have. You helped me learn how to enjoy myself.'

Before we met, my familial combination of Scottish Presbyterianism and English Methodism had resulted in a somewhat spartan way of life. I am still too hard on myself but now I weigh the benefits and hazards of my own lifestyle, just like I used to help my patients to do.

'I don't want you to make changes for me,' says John, 'I want you to do it for you.'

I have wondered about coming off the antidepressants completely, a change I would like to make. After broaching the subject with my psychiatrist in hospital, I withdrew from one of them successfully. Now I began again, 'Sometime soon, I'm not sure when but it will probably be the end of next year ... I think ... I hope ... we will be moving North. Will you make a referral for me to another specialist up there?'

He looked a little surprised that I was thinking so many months ahead, but I needed to know. 'Yes, of course,' he said.

'And maybe I could cut down the tablets ... eventually?' How many times had patients asked me this?

We both knew the answer, but I had asked anyway. 'Perhaps... Let's see how things go. It's probably a little too soon with all that has been happening for you.'

He was right. If I were to cut down when my life was going through upheaval, as it is at the moment, there would be a risk of relapse. I have seen many patients weaned (how I hate that infantilising term) off medication when the stresses haven't gone away. I will never forget meeting the parents of a young man who had come off his tablets after finishing university and starting a high-pressure job a long way from home. His new doctor was unaware of the severity of his previous episode and didn't explore how much stress he was still under. A couple of months later that young man took his life.

'We wanted to talk to someone, to try and understand why it happened ... ' his father said. 'Our GP recommended that we come and talk to you.'

I did my best to answer their questions. 'Sometimes it just isn't the right time to make a change in medication.'

'He was very worried about it,' his mother said. 'He was

still having to cope with a great deal, but he had been feeling well and just wanted to put it all behind him.'

'He wasn't sure what to do but, in the end, he stopped,' his father added. 'We wondered if it was the right thing to do, but the new doctor said that six months was long enough to be on them.' Perhaps not for this person at this time in his life. There are no hard rules. It isn't so uncommon, and when it happens it is tragic, because it is so preventable.

Given the kind of medication I am on, the high dose, and the very long time that I've been taking the tablets, withdrawal symptoms would be highly likely. The only solution would be to come off them very slowly indeed.

'I don't think you should stop them,' says John. 'I've seen you on them, and off them, and I would worry.'

The hope of one day being medication-free is strong. There is something about taking tablets for the mind that differs from my other medication, because of how they change what it means to be yourself. You question your authenticity. 'Am I now a different person from who I was before I took the tablets? If I come off them, who is then the real me?

Christmas has passed and we are walking to the shore of Loch of Stenness, not far from the house. Behind us loom the remaining Neolithic stones of the Ring of Brodgar, which have been standing here in the centre of Mainland Orkney for five thousand years. No-one knows why it was built or for what purpose, but it must have had spiritual significance when the climate was warmer than it is now. During the summer hordes of tourists disgorge at the car park and walk the circular path around the great monoliths before heading back to their coaches.

In the evening, when everyone has gone and the mist closes in, or on winter days like this when the sun shines cold and clear for an hour or two, I sometimes have a sixth sense of the flow of life – past and present – just as I did among the totems in Haida Gwaii.

There must be such magical sites in the South too, but I do not know them, and I suspect they wouldn't hold the same fascination for me. We must all find our own special places.

This is one of our favourite walks when the days are short and the sun begins to set over the hills of Hoy. The water of the loch turns from blue to a shimmering silver as the sky closes in behind us and we can visualise the sun streaming into the entrance chamber of Maeshowe, a Neolithic tomb nearby, lighting up the interior as it does every Winter Solstice.

'You haven't talked very much about your mother.' Opening on this subject isn't easy, 'I know I've been away quite a lot this last couple of months when I should have been with you. I'm so sorry.'

John squeezes my hand. He is on the edge of tears. 'I feel so lost now that she is gone. I'm not sure where my life is going.'

We again talk about him coming to live here permanently. This is a place where I feel I can create something, a place to be that would give my life meaning, but I can see he is much less sure.

'I know how much this means to you...' he begins.

The air is chilling fast. We turn back up the hill, kicking holes in the ice with our heels. The stones are silhouetted against the sky, looming in the gathering darkness, and the power that comes with their antiquity and what they have witnessed across the millennia is almost palpable.

This place feels more like 'home' than anywhere I have lived in the last four decades, since leaving my place of birth, but maybe I am in danger of investing too much in it. I've wanted to return North all my life, but if it isn't right for John, my partner in life, then perhaps I must let go of that dream. Viktor Frankl was right, above all we find our meaning in life through love, and the love between us has been so important in sustaining me over the last thirty years.

There are many risks to investing in the love of another. They may let you down, reject you or simply die. Painful experience can mean that we avoid taking those risks again, stay 'safe', keep our distance and avoid depending on anyone but ourselves. But loving and being loved makes us more aware of our own potential to find renewed hope and meaning in life.

My husband is grieving, and I must help him.

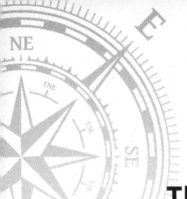

CHAPTER 10

The problem with forgiveness

Memories charged with emotion linger. More than forty years ago, I took the bus from Stromness to Kirkwall, down the chain of linked southern islands to South Ronaldsay, past the splendid Italian Chapel, to the southernmost village of St Margaret's Hope. Then, as now, was a time of fear, but also hope. Of leaving one home and searching for another.

Bathed in the pure light of the vast Northern sky, the vista of land and water still takes my breath away as we drive over the hill. Swans return year after year to rear their cygnets. Seals sometimes loll in the shallows by the Brig O'Waithe, or swim further into the loch to pose on the rocks near the Standing Stones. Otters must live here too, but as a late riser I never see them. The homes and farms of other Orcadians are scattered across the landscape. Sometimes the water is calm, and the hills picked out in reflections like the bold brush strokes of an old master, only to disappear as the sky turns to grey and the wind whips 'white horses' across the loch. Other times, like today as we drive through a swirling haar back to the house, the view possesses the qualities of an unfinished watercolour, still awash with pale and translucent hues. In common with their inhabitants, landscapes are always changing and evolving.

'What's the plan for this morning?' John asks. 'Are we going out?'

'I'd like to get something done on writing about my journey back to Lincolnshire. Can we go later? For lunch?'

'You look settled down to work.'

At my desk, where there is now not only my mug of pens and pencils but another for paintbrushes that I am not yet quite ready to use. Sometimes only writing can make sense of our experiences.

It was a month after New Year when I drove over the toll bridge on the River Trent from Yorkshire into Lincolnshire. As though to herald my homecoming to the English county that most wanted to turn back time by leaving the European Union, and where I grew up, five Red Arrow jets, based nearby, flew overhead in perfect formation.

Next morning found me wandering as though in a daze. Having so often travelled back to this place during sleep, checking into the hotel where I'd once been an underage drinker seemed surreal. Most of the shops in Skegness had changed. Others were frozen in time with the surnames of people I had been to school with still above the doors. The geography was changed almost in the same way that it is in dreams. The familiar juxtaposed with the unexpected. I learned how to drive many years after I left home. So, finding my way around from behind the wheel of a car only added to my sense of dislocation.

The bus station had been transformed into a pizza

restaurant. Marks and Spencer's in the main street, where I worked on Saturdays on the checkout till, was a bargain store. Along the road in what was once the Co-op, the first escalator that I ever stepped onto as a small child still travelled up to the first floor. The amusement park, with its giant switchback 'Figure Eight', where my father worked when I was young, had been razed and only a tarmacked car park remained. It was here where he collected, from between the tracks, silver threepenny pieces people had lost when paying for their rides. He attached them to a silver bracelet for me.

After walking down the broad avenue where I lived for the first eighteen years of my life, I stood in front of my childhood home. It still had two bay windows and one front door but there were three doorbells now, not one. This house, in this small town, was my hermetically sealed world for almost the first third of my life, confining me as though in a snow globe. It was more than thirty years since I had escaped.

Memories flood my mind. When difficult things have happened in my life, things that challenged my fragile sense of self – the end of a relationship, criticism from a colleague – I have experienced, at times, a sudden shift in mood to one of excruciating anguish. My behaviour has been alarming, even to those who have been willing to stick around. Destructive anger and a terrible feeling of emptiness so powerful that the very heart of me, this 'self' that I have worked so hard to create, could be smashed forever. In our household, people lashed out in anger. My mother slapped me, but when my father used his giant calloused working man's hand it was much more painful, both physically and emotionally. The problems in my relationships originated in that house and live there with the ghosts of my past, which is why I needed to go back.

I hadn't set out that morning to find my mother's grave, but soon realised it was a visit long overdue. Walking up and down the rows in the cemetery for half an hour I found the section for the people of Skegness buried in the autumn of 2012, the year she died. It took some time to find her name. Looking for a headstone I found only a small wooden cross with a fading metal plaque. She would have been disappointed that no-one erected an elaborate memorial in her memory.

In the decade before her death we had almost no contact. The last time I saw her was around the turn of the millennium, when John and I were attempting to build bridges with her and her partner of thirty years. She had been having treatment for breast cancer and travelling a long distance across the county for radiotherapy. During our visit she developed pain in her leg and had difficulty breathing but was reluctant to call the GP. I examined her as best I could.

'I really think you must call the doctor.'

'I don't want to bother them,' she insisted, in that accent which sounded Scottish in England, and English in Scotland.

'I mean it, I think this is serious.'

Later that day she was taken into hospital with blood clots on the lung. By insisting she saw the doctor I had possibly saved her life. We spoke on the telephone after she had made her recovery, but then lost touch again. Every time I heard her voice it triggered a mixture of anger, loneliness and, finally, simple sadness. I didn't realise it, but I had been grieving for my mother for many years and, unlike John, for the mother I never had.

Almost six years ago my youngest brother Graeme, with whom I've had very little contact in the last forty years, telephoned to tell me that our mother had died of lung cancer. She had been ill for only four weeks. It was a quick but horrible way to die, with relentless coughing and gasping for breath. I didn't attend the funeral. My mother blamed me for much of her unhappiness for reasons I never fully understood, and my remaining family seemed to share that view. Was it because we had so little contact, or because I wasn't the child she wanted? I suspect the latter.

My mother did not love me. Jumbled images of the past come and go and with them the emotions of anger, hurt and sadness that I talked about with my therapists. I hadn't felt her love, but what I did experience was resentment, jealousy, anger and ridicule. There is a scene that replays in my head, because it was recorded on film and we watched it regularly, sometimes with people outside the immediate family. I was eleven years old. We were on holiday in Devon and my father had bought a second-hand cine camera as it was our first real family holiday. My mother climbed a children's slide, and as she came down her dress blew up. I ran over to hold it down.

'Oh, look at her! Such a prude and a wee bit of a snob too.' She laughed at me at the time and on every occasion we watched it, telling everyone present exactly what she thought of me. I blushed until my face was sore. Every time the Kodak projector came out of its box, I dreaded the moment she approached the slide and felt repeatedly humiliated.

Sometimes our families do not value the qualities that make us unique, but instead criticise and mock us for them. My mother derided me repeatedly in many ways, some subtle, others less so. I slowly grew to hate myself.

John brings me a cup of tea and my favourite treat, a dark chocolate Tunnock's caramel wafer. 'Have a break.'

'Graeme said that I look so much like Mum.' There are tears in my eyes. My brother, who is still in the army, got in touch a couple of years ago, and we met in London, for the first time in decades.

'You aren't like her at all. I only met her a couple of times, when she was ill, but I couldn't see anything of her in you.'

'I can. Her determination to survive.'

We know so much more now about the effect of adverse childhood experiences. The persisting effects on the mind and body: difficulties with mood, behaviour, ability to make relationships and function in the world. Physical symptoms that cannot be explained, but do not go away. Problems that not only contribute to failures of recovery but also result in a diagnosis of personality disorder. People who have lived through trauma do not recover quickly. How could they? A few half hour sessions with a therapist is not a magic bullet.

During my last few years at work in Salford, I supervised young therapists. One afternoon, when we had gathered in a stifling hot first floor room during a summer heatwave to discuss patients, Anna, who had just rushed in, began, 'This morning, two people out of the five who were booked in to see me told me they had been abused in childhood. I mean people do disclose things sometimes, but this morning ... it felt too much ...'

'Too much to cope with ...?'

Anna was flushed. I wasn't sure whether it was simply the heat, or the intensity of emotion, both the patients' and her own. 'I feel a bit guilty saying that. I mean ... I've heard awful things before, but today ...'

'Sometimes it's hard to listen... why don't you join us and then we can discuss the best way to try and help?'

'But what can we offer people in the time we have?' She sounded exhausted.

'Let's start from the beginning . . . tell us something about the first person you saw today.' Learning how to be with and hear people talk about traumatic experiences is tough. We did the best we could in difficult circumstances as services were being cut back. In supervising others, I drew on all my experience as a psychiatrist, a teacher and as a patient myself, to try and hold everyone together.

I didn't experience the major traumas that many of our patients endured, but without secure, loving parental attachments when we are fearful and distressed, lesser traumas are quite damaging enough.[12] We don't develop a healthy sense of self-esteem. Years after I left home and was going through divorce from my first husband, struggling to keep my life together, I spoke to my mother on the telephone.

'Why did you get married in such a rush?' Actually, I had been twenty-two, older than she was when she married my father, but still a medical student.

'Because I didn't think anyone else would want me.' I had always known that somewhere inside but, only after years of therapy, could I say it aloud to her.

'You shouldn't have thought that.' For a moment she sounded genuinely shocked. Had she really not known how little self-esteem I possessed?

It was too late to repair the damage.

John puts his hand on my shoulder.

'The sun is shining. Shall we get out for a walk? I think you need a break.'

'Can I just have a little longer?' I say. 'Half an hour?'

He is trying to get me away from my desk to escape my head and spend some time in the real world with him. The problem is that the past can sometimes feel just as real as the present.

Perhaps, as children, we learn to hide our feelings to try and win the love of our parents. We survive by repressing who we really are and may not want to admit that our childhood wasn't 'happy'. It may only be in therapy that we acknowledge what happened. How our parents treat us is often a reflection of what they experienced in their own childhoods. There is a vicious cycle at work.

My mother had been a survivor of a difficult childhood too. Her own mother had fallen unconscious in the street when they were out together and died soon after. Mum was only twelve years old. She never talked about it but losing a parent when you are young is a risk factor in adult mental health problems.

It must have been a tough existence. Three children on their own, with a miner for a father, who died only a few years later from the last gasps of the 1940s tuberculosis epidemic, not long before effective antibiotics were discovered. A couple of years ago, on my way through Lanarkshire, I re-visited the streets where she had brought me as a child only to find that, unsurprisingly, everything looked different. In my memory, where images are frozen in time, the old Whitehill council estate hadn't changed at all. Seeing the modern doors and windows in the houses and green spaces where ugly tenements had once stood, enabled me to begin moving on from my past.

What, I wonder, had Mum's relationship been like with

the stern looking man wearing an Orange sash[13] whom I only know from creased and curling black and white photographs kept in an old shoebox? Was he kind or harsh? Did he expect her to be the daughter that later she wanted me to be, giving up school and getting a job? I know he washed in a tin bath in front of the fire, but he also baked the family cakes every week, just as I did as a teenager. The pits and their 'bings' were disappearing even when I was young and have now been thoroughly landscaped away into history.

Returning to significant places can be important. People who experience stressful events may avoid places for years, even a lifetime, yet it can be helpful to bear witness that the world has moved beyond that which haunts you.

Once, having returned from a trip to Mostar in Bosnia-Herzegovina, where I had watched young men dive from the famous bridge that was rebuilt after the Balkan war, an ex-serviceman who had served there more than a decade before came into my clinic. He was haunted by what he had witnessed – the horror of ethnic cleansing. He could not believe that I had just been there too, as a tourist.

'Can I see your photographs?' he asked.

Cautiously I agreed, concerned about triggering his distress with images that might transport him back in time. Yet he was able to appreciate the difference between the past and the present.

My trauma had been nothing like his, yet I needed to go back again too. I wanted to see how the places of my child-hood had changed, and not have distorted memories forever invade my dreams.

*

'I wish I could forgive her,' I say to John.

'Do you have to?'

As we trudge along the path on the north mainland at the Brough of Birsay, waves roll over ancient slabs of rock and the air tastes of salt and seaweed. We often walk here. Sometimes there are seals hauled up on the rocks, but not today. It isn't the kind of longer march that John would prefer, but it's enough for an afternoon stroll, and especially energising when the wind is blowing towards you. We are heading towards the weathered whale bone sculpture that someone, probably more than a century ago, erected on the headland near Skipi Geo. There are different theories for how it came to be here. A whale came ashore on the beach. It was probably already dead when it washed up. But why create this structure from its skull and jawbone? No one knows.

Many whose lives have been blighted by what has happened to them in childhood cannot understand or forgive and continue to fight for justice. Anger and pain propel them. In *On Forgiveness*, Richard Holloway talks about the need to separate the person from the act. A terrible act must not be forgiven, he says, otherwise we lose our ability to distinguish between right and wrong. We must try and forgive the person behind the act if we are to take back agency in our lives.

Yet forgiveness never comes easily. For me it was complicated by how my mother sought to blame someone else for my later problems with my mental health. I've told John this several times, but he still listens as I recount the latest discovery in the saga. Two decades ago, I discovered that my paternal grandfather, who had lived with us when I was a child, spent six months in prison. All this had happened not long before I was born.

'I did tell you what I found out about Grandpa, didn't I? It was a newspaper report of an appeal against conviction for indecent assault on five young girls, all children. It was all there, in the library.'

'Mum says she feels guilty because Grandpa might have done something to you too,' my brother Alan told me on the phone years ago. 'That's why you might have these problems . . . she didn't do anything to stop it.'

'But he didn't.' I insisted. At least I didn't remember anything. Some will say *but you might not remember it* but by this time I had been in therapy on and off for years. 'Grandma never believed it. She refused to, but everyone else knew.'

So much that had puzzled me about my childhood began to slot into place. My grandmother's powerful mistrust of anyone outside the family. 'Why do you have to bring them back here?' she would ask, when I brought my school friends home. The curious lack of respect that some members of the family seemed to have for Grandpa. 'I really don't have to do anything he tells me to,' my uncle's wife would say when Grandpa shouted at her. A cynical disdain that I can now put a name to. That my grandparents never went to chapel despite having been brought up strict Methodists. Grandma spent her days playing hymns on the piano. They wouldn't have attended, because that was where the events that became our great family secret took place, a stone's throw from our house, which my grandparents had once run as a seaside hotel.

I discovered that old copies of the local newspaper were available in the local library and went there on the afternoon of my arrival in Skegness. Grandpa and I spent hours rooting around these shelves in my early childhood. Once when I read both my books in a day, I asked him to take me back in the early evening before they closed. He sighed, 'We can't take books back the same day because they have to move all those tickets on the front desk around at night, it would cause confusion.' I always believed him.

More than half a century later, when I expected to find only microfiche copies of the *Skegness Standard*, I was surprised when the library assistant brought out a large binder of original newsprint, faded to brown and with the damp scent of age. A brief search located the report of his trial from July 1951:

> '*Hotelier sent to gaol: guilty plea to serious charges was the only good thing.*'

My beloved grandfather, with whom I had spent day after day as an only child before the birth of my brothers, had pleaded guilty to three counts of indecent assault on girls between the ages of eight and twelve, and asked for two other offences to be taken into consideration. Five girls. Our next-door neighbour, who spoke as a character witness on my grandfather's behalf had been so shocked that his 'emotions overcame him' while speaking to the bench. '*He (witness) had girls of his own and they had been in company of accused.*' As a child I played with the neighbour's youngest daughter.

Grandpa was sentenced to six months in prison. Today it would be much longer.

Had he done anything similar before? Did he repeat it? Experience tells me that the answers to both might be 'yes'. There was a letter from his doctor about treatment for an undisclosed health problem. Had he been under stress, or am

I simply trying to find excuses for him? Would I have been able to forgive if I was one of those children or mothers? No, but there was nothing untoward about his behaviour towards me. He had once run a business selling sewing machines. When I was young, both he and my father still did the occasional repair. That was how one of the girls had known who he was, because he had repaired her mother's machine. Later, he worked for years as a travelling salesman and I went everywhere with him in his van to collect hire purchase payments from farmers' wives. It was a great adventure for me.

My bedroom was at the top of the house next to the one he shared with my grandmother. I was eleven years old and sleeping next door on the morning he awoke with slight discomfort in his chest. 'Make us a cup of tea will you, Ev?' he said to her. Her name was Evelyn. Those were his last words. When she returned he had passed away. He was the first person that I had loved or even known who had died.

'He must have been ill,' I tell John. 'Perhaps he was depressed. Maybe he had an alcohol problem.' There had always been empty bottles of rum and brandy under the kitchen sink. He drank it with his tea, but like a good Methodist, had always told me that it was 'for medicinal purposes only'.

'Why? Perhaps that is just who he was, but sometimes we can't make sense of things however hard we try. You should know that better than anyone.'

I should, but it doesn't stop me making excuses for him in my head.

Now we are back at the house, John has lit the stove and we have retreated to the kitchen to prepare for dinner.

'What's that?' he asks, as I unwrap a paper bag.

'It's a fridge magnet, I bought it in Skegness.' Small scenes of the favourite place of my childhood, Gibraltar Point, where I went for long walks with my father.

One summer evening, when I was in my mid-teens, I had come downstairs in a new black halter neck maxi dress which revealed more of me than usual, although I had covered my red sunburned shoulders with a generous dusting of talcum powder stuck on with body lotion. I had been out all day at Gibraltar Point in the hot sunshine for a geography field course, counting the number of times a plant could be found in each square metre of salt marsh, but foolishly hadn't taken any sun cream. Before I could get to the front door Dad emerged from the lounge with a: 'You aren't going out in that, are you?'

My terse affirmation was met with a frown of disapproval. I wondered what was wrong with my appearance, confidence sapping away. Did I look a mess? Did the dress make me look ugly? We were as stubborn as each other, but he didn't try to stop me when I opened the front door and stepped out.

'Don't be late!' he called after me. I didn't look back.

On this last visit to the Point once again, this time bathed in January sunshine, I went for my prescribed daily brisk walk, along the familiar track between the salt marsh and sparkling ponds. It was impossible to reach the grey-blue waters of the Wash, now sprouting giant alien-like wind turbines, because the creek that crossed the beach was too deep and I didn't have wellies with me. Waves pounded the shore as I stood on top of the sand dunes, under a vast clear blue sky, looking out to sea. Later, I sat drinking my morning Americano in the new visitor centre, where you can idly watch the birdlife. When I had come here with Dad there had rarely been anyone except birdwatchers, even in the high season. Now the car park was full, and you had to 'pay and display'. He would have hated it because there were too many people and it was no longer wild and free. I was ambivalent, wanting both freedom and the good coffee too.

'There was a man selling postcards and guidebooks who looked about my age,' I tell John, 'but he didn't seem to recognise me.'

'It's more than forty years since you left.'

I pull a face and laugh. 'Anyway, that's where I bought this. I don't know why. It's just a souvenir.'

'I stayed here all week once,' I said to the man I might have known, pointing through the vast glass window to the old coastguard station, 'for a biology field trip.'

'You couldn't do that now.' I smiled, thinking he meant because I was older now, but he carried on. 'You see it's all gone at the rear now, just the old building still standing. The wooden bit got swept away in the big storm a couple of years back.'

'Gosh, I remember that night.' I had followed on the internet how my hometown had been threatened, just as in the Great Flood in 1952 when hundreds died in the countries surrounding the North Sea.

'Water was right up to here,' he gestured to his waist. We were already well above ground level and I could see why the new centre had been elevated.

It was strangely satisfying. Whatever we build, however we get above ourselves in life, the ocean has a curious way of bringing everything into perspective.

Later that day I found myself once again in a cemetery. Or rather the garden of remembrance at the crematorium in

Boston, where my father's ashes had been scattered. I'd often thought of returning but never felt able. For many years I'd failed to grieve, and even after acknowledging my yearning for the father whose love had been my saving grace, I still couldn't do it. Now I had come, but it was a month too late to see his name in the Book of Remembrance and the cabinet was locked. After trying to open it I looked around to see a CCTV camera pointing directly at me. I wandered out instead among the rose bushes, pausing now and then to read the names on the tags attached to the stems before the tears began to flow and I sobbed aloud.

I will never fully understand why my father and I grew apart, but my mother's relationship with me played a large part. She stirred up anger between us by complaining about me to him at every opportunity. Much older, and hopefully wiser, I can see that how I behaved towards her must have hurt him because he loved her. I shouted and screamed at him in anger, and there were times when he hit me hard. My terrible feelings of pain and unbearable shame originate in the minutes and hours I cried myself to sleep. The red marks took time to fade, but not as long as the emotions.

If you carry a memory of having felt safe with someone long ago, traces of that earlier affection can be reactivated later, whether in therapy or real life. To grow up with insecure attachments is to start adult life at a disadvantage, but many things can happen to impact positively on our trajectories. Not least the nurturing love of a therapist or a partner.

I have been fortunate to have both.

Some say that therapists shouldn't tell us to forgive because we need to remember and re-experience our childhood pain.

However, getting in touch with those powerful emotions can be extraordinarily difficult and take many years.

My father was a complex man, anxious, irritable, disappointed in life and difficult to please. Through long hours of therapy, I came to understand that he had loved me, but that, growing older, we found it impossible to express our feelings. I wish he had lived long enough to talk about the past and make peace.

My mother always told us how she missed her family, but I doubt she fitted into that dark Lanarkshire landscape any more than I did. Was that why she left to travel south, only a few months older than I was when I first came here to Orkney? Prematurely widowed, she embraced a very different life: enjoying her first holidays in the sun, an invitation to a garden party at Buckingham Palace, and wearing a huge diamond ring on her finger from her new partner. The quarter century she spent with my father struggling to make ends meet must have seemed like another lifetime. When she died, I felt very little sorrow as my grieving for her had long been done. In seeking to put the blame for my mental health problems on my grandfather, she had sought to be a victim rather than a perpetrator, which is why it is so hard for me to forgive. It was always about *her* being let down by her husband's family. Even after death I can still sense the rivalry for my father's attention and concern.

'Your mother loved you very much,' I say to John as we sit in the glow of the fire. The wind has whipped up again, and two more stormy days are forecast.

'Sometimes it felt like too much ... no, I shouldn't say that. I know how much she cared about me.'

'And you her. You couldn't have done any more for her than you did. You do know that, don't you?'

The worst of the storm has passed. According to the weather forecast, we are probably somewhere near the eye, and more wind and rain is expected, but for the moment we can get to Stromness to go shopping without being bent double by the gale. If someone asked what the colour of the Orkney sky is today, you might only reply 'blue and grey', but that would be an understatement, because there are so many different hues that I could recreate by mixing together white with varying amounts of raw umber and ultramarine on my painter's palette.

'I love the skies here, they are so huge and complex,' I say.

'That's why I like photographing them, but don't they remind you of home?'

'I've never thought of that.'

The place where I come from, the Lincolnshire salt marsh, is completely flat. Orkney has low hills but so much space from which to watch the skies. I am situated between sea and sky, despite having always wanted to escape to the mountains.

'I remember when you took me to Gibraltar Point,' he says. 'The sky was so vast. It was almost impossible to do it justice.' His images captured the haunting loneliness around the fringes of The Wash. 'Maybe that's one of the reasons you love it here so much.'

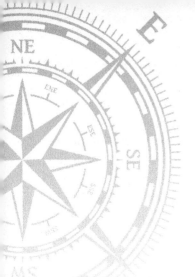

CHAPTER 11

Healing

Although we hardly see the sun, each day now is almost imperceptibly longer than the one before. Yesterday, in the periphery of my vision, I glimpsed a hare through the window in the garden, but when I looked up it had gone. If I wasn't mistaken, it was my first sighting this year. Spring will soon be with us again.

The last time we returned to Orkney it was dark when we drove off the ferry. Only scattered lights were visible as we came over the hill from Stromness, but then, as we rounded the loch, a greenish band of light appeared across the Northern sky. I didn't take much note of it, having just come from South Yorkshire where the sky is always so polluted with light from the cities. However, as I was carrying in bags from the car, John called to me, 'Come outside quick and see the sky!'

At that moment, Mary from the farm pulled up beside us in her car. We hugged. 'Can you see the Mirrie Dancers?' she asked, pointing to the North. That's what they call the Aurora Borealis in the Northern Isles. And here they were, in all their shimmering glory – veils of green and yellow light moving and shifting as the gowns of ethereal performers swept around the sky.

Despite many visits to the North, I had never managed to see the Aurora. When camping in Iceland many years ago, one member of our group decided to sleep outside his tent, probably to show us all how tough were part-time soldiers in the Swiss army. Next morning, he casually informed everyone that he had seen the Northern Lights whilst lying awake, staring at the cold night sky. 'I didn't want to wake any of you,' he said. The rest of us hadn't been sure whether to believe him or not.

More recently, on a journey to Arkhangelsk in northern Russia in the darkness of mid-winter, when the Dvina was frozen solid from bank to bank, I watched the northern sky every night hoping to see them, but the dancers never appeared, even though that city is a good deal further north than Orkney. The Norwegians travelling with us laughed at me and boasted, 'You should come to Tromsø. We see them all the time!'

Not long ago, Mary told me she'd been out to the barn the night before, seeing to the cows, and had looked up to see them shimmering in the sky. 'We have them here sometimes,' she said, 'You have to be outside at the right time.'

'When it happens again, call me please whatever time it is!' I begged.

However, that night in March we had been in the right place, at the right time. We stood gazing towards the horizon until our faces were numb in the cold night air, and the celestial show had all but finished.

'Perhaps it's a good omen,' John said, and pulled me close.

I don't believe in magic, but I do believe in magical moments – those occasions when something special happens – even mystical things. When we marvel at natural phenomena, like an extraordinary sunrise, the golden light of the gloaming, or the Aurora, which is truly out of this world. At other times the stimulus for that sense of wonder isn't obvious, but you don't have to be religious to acknowledge the spiritual element of our existence and recognise how humanity can transcend the certainties of life.

Sometimes interactions between human beings possess a singular power. When, for the first time in your life, you connect with another person and find someone who seems to understand you. When, as an adult you realise something you never felt in childhood, that there is someone who really does love you, regardless of the baggage you carry from the past. When you experience forgiveness from another for something you still can't forgive yourself for. When you allow yourself to believe there is another way to live your life and it isn't all predestined. These times hold the essence of emotional healing and are magical too.

'You are really very well at the moment,' John says, 'I don't think I've seen you so consistently well in years.'

'I am,' I smile and say, 'but I'm not sure why.'

That isn't entirely true. Something is happening. I'm rebuilding my life and beginning to find meaning in existence again.

The sun is streaming into the kitchen window, raising our spirits, but the forecast says it will not last. People often say about island weather that if you don't like the current conditions you only have to wait half an hour. But clouds are gathering, and the needle of the old brass barometer in the window of the diving shop in Stromness was dropping when I saw it earlier this morning. There is a storm on its way.

One December, not long after I first moved into the Wee Hoose, I flew into Kirkwall through a 'weather bomb' that had encroached on northern Scotland. It was calm when we left Aberdeen, but soon the wind began to buffet the plane violently, not only from side to side but also up and down. Descending towards the islands we turned on a dipped wing into a curve, a familiar holding pattern.

'Sorry about this everyone,' came the calm voice of the co-pilot, 'there's a snowstorm at the airport so it's going to be a while before we can make our approach.'

For the next fifteen minutes, although it could have been longer, we jerked through troughs and peaks of stormy grey, with the flinty surface of the sea occasionally illuminated by lightning flashes. I shared a false smile with a woman across the aisle, one of the three other brave passengers who hadn't changed their travel plans. It was terrifying, but the disembodied voice of the co-pilot was reassuring. 'Ladies and gentlemen, I know it's been a difficult flight, but you'll be pleased to know they have just checked the runway. It's safe and we'll have you on the ground in a few minutes.'

Storms arrive here every winter. Sometimes the telephone is cut off, the mobile phone mast fails and the fields flood. As the climate changes, the islands are experiencing greater extremes of weather, yet there is something special about living here in closer harmony with nature. You cannot escape from the sky – wherever you are it is always visible, demanding you take account of it. It can be harsh and may seem too grey and judgemental at times, but can suddenly surprise you with the bright, clear midwinter sunshine that reminds you how much closer we are to Scandinavia than southern England.

Like the weather, my moods can change suddenly. When I've been depressed it has often felt as if the evil controller in my brain has pulled a lever. Within hours I can shift from feeling anxious, but keeping my head above water, to quite a different state of mind. Not only sad but physically changed. Heavy of limb, tired, unable to sleep, yet also agitated and fearful as negative thoughts about myself, the world and the future flood back. It hasn't happened for a while, but I suspect depression has not left me for good. That isn't me being pessimistic, just realistic.

A few months ago, some of my tablets were changed because my blood pressure was still too high, even though I was taking a full dose of medication. 'The renal people like to keep it within very tight limits,' my GP told me, but I already knew that. I had been reading up about it on the internet as usual.

'This is what I usually try next.' In addition to the existing pills she started me on another one.

'When I was put on those, my ankles nearly swelled up to my knees,' a fellow psychiatrist I've known since medical school told me in Edinburgh not long after. Retired doctors share their illness stories over dinner just like everyone else.

At first everything was fine. My blood pressure came down to the desired level, but after a few weeks my joints began to ache all the time and my mood, so buoyant for months, suddenly began to slide for no apparent reason.

John noticed as always, 'Something isn't right, is it?' I

had been in tears at the thought of him going away for a couple of days, something neither of us could understand.

'No . . . I've started to have thoughts that life isn't worth living again, and I'm frightened.'

My psychiatrist made the connection between mood and medication quickly. 'I've seen this several times before. I think you have to come off the new pills but see your GP again and find out if there's anything else you can take. Keeping your blood pressure low may be best, but not at the cost of your mental health.'

Within a few days of stopping, I was considerably better in mind and body, and before long back to where I had been. I'm now taking another type which seems to work well without causing the same problems. It's been an enormous relief.

Stresses in life may trigger a relapse of depression. There are always uncertainties on the horizon. A little while ago we discovered there are plans to build a new electricity substation nearby in this part of Mainland. Orkney is a hub for green energy development, especially wave and wind power, harnessing the tidal surges in the Pentland Firth and some of the most powerful winds in Western Europe. The network apparently needs to be modernised to cope with the increase in generating capacity as more huge wind turbines come on-line. There's been a great deal of debate in the letter column of *The Orcadian*. Some people saying that it is essential that the islands do their bit for tackling global warming, and others that the plans are simply unacceptable. Everyone is concerned whether the new developments can happen in a way that is sympathetic to the landscape and heritage of these islands.

'How is this going to affect our plans?' John asks.

'Should it?' We've started planning a permanent move to Orkney even though John still isn't sure that it is right for him. Nothing is fixed.

'Maybe we should look around for other possibilities ... '

One option would be to stay in England. Although I love it, for me, the north of England will always be associated with work. Towns and cities where I spent my life meeting others' needs. Another alternative is to look for somewhere a little further south on the Scottish Mainland. John knows my preference has always been for him to move here to live with me, but I'm trying not to push him into making a hasty decision.

I say, 'I'm older than you, I'm in my mid-sixties already, I guess I just feel ready to settle somewhere fairly soon, not spend the next few years searching for the perfect place.' Somewhere that probably doesn't exist, because I'm beginning to realise that achieving peace of mind isn't only about the physical place in which we live, but about how we feel in ourselves. We create a healing space inside of us.

'I know what you mean,' he says, 'The journeys are getting more tiring aren't they?' We both miss having animal companions too. We need to live in one place, either here or in the south if we are to give a home to another cat.

The aim of therapy is the development of a more reflective, independent 'self', which can come to feel like a healthy 'island' within all the chaos reflected in our lives. However, that doesn't only happen within therapy, and the processes of self-reflection and gradual understanding can continue over many years. Being able to tell your own story, in your own way, to someone who will listen without judgment, or perhaps to write it down, can be important. Your 'healthy island' grows within you, as your mind and body begin to heal.

Just as it takes time and effort to preserve and cherish the unique beauty of these islands, looking after ourselves can be hard work. There are things that we can do to lessen the impact that stress has on our lives but we need the support, care and patience of others.

'You're very high performance,' John tells me, using his favourite racing car analogy, 'but you easily go out of tune. You need a lot of tender, loving care.'

The psychiatrist who has taken care of me for the last few years is unable to continue, so I will no longer have his support to fall back on if I need it.

'The service is closing,' he told me last time I went to see him.

'I don't understand why. Surely there is a demand for better quality care for people with depression?' Those who don't feel any improvement at all after years of different treatment or, like me, wax and wane in our moods. Those of us who struggle with the idea that 'depression' is no more than 'feeling sad', when we know that what we are experiencing isn't just about what is going on in the world, or even in our heads, but affects our entire physical being.

'The NHS doesn't want to pay for it, that's the problem,' he explained, although I knew that already. People are expected to get better with brief therapy, or maybe medication, but the zeitgeist is moving away from taking tablets because of the problems they cause for some people, even though for others with more severe depression, like me, they really do help. Longer term therapy is much harder to access these days too without paying.

Like physical wounds, psychological ones need the right

therapy and conditions in which to heal and can leave deep scars. The expectations of brief therapy and medication are similar, to kick-start your mind or your body to take up life again, but a simple 'fix' doesn't work for everyone. We keep hearing how, someday, there will be medication tailored to suit each individual, but I don't think there will ever be a tablet labelled 'take two a day to come to terms with how you feel about your mother.'

We discussed the possibility of my seeing someone else privately, but I declined. Getting to know someone gradually, over time, and building trust in them, has always been important to me. There's little value in being 'assessed' by one health professional after another because you never get a chance to build up a relationship with them – and that is a powerful part of treatment. As a doctor, I was the person who was the 'keeper' of my patients' stories. They didn't have to repeat their story every time they consulted me. It feels too much of an effort to start that process with someone new, all over again.

'I'm really very well at the moment,' I tell him. 'I will see how it goes from here.'

'I will write,' he says, 'and send a summary that might help if you want to see someone else and . . . ' He holds out his hand, 'I'm so pleased to have been able to take care of you.'

I am working with a group of people from voluntary organisations in Orkney, discussing how to help people cope with bereavement and grief. It's a topic I have returned to so often, both during my career and my own life. We are gathered in a top floor room in an old building in Kirkwall near the harbour that looks, from the black and white photographs around the wall, to have a fascinating history, originally as some kind of workshop. Except we are at work today with our minds rather than our hands. There are half a dozen people with me, and everyone is engaged.

'We underestimate how difficult grief can be for some people,' I say. 'If you've had a complicated relationship with the dead person it is especially hard. A couple of years ago, someone I shared the stage with at a Science Festival, a neuroscientist, started to talk about grieving for the loss of an active lifestyle after he had a serious cycling accident. I'm not sure he had realised he had been grieving until he heard me speaking about the impact of loss.'

It had been a curious moment. One of those times when people from very different ends of the psychological spectrum suddenly find a connection. He talked with candour about how he had, with time, managed to get himself going again. I doubt he had expected to be sharing that kind of story when we walked on stage.

'However, when you lose someone about whom you have ambivalent feelings, it can be so much more difficult to work through your grief and emerge from the other side.' We get stuck. We hold onto the pain, the anger and despair inside us, and do not let go of it. Eventually that turns into something rather like depression, but medication alone isn't sufficient.

'We have to talk about what happened and gradually let go of the past while re-engaging with life and beginning to make new memories.'

Most of that happened many years ago for me, in therapy, but I had always avoided returning to the crematorium to say goodbye. Almost forty years later, I finally did. After the session, one of the group, a chaplain from the hospital whom

I'd met at a previous event, asks me if we can have a chat.

'What are you doing now?'

'Well, I'm no longer working as a psychiatrist,' I reply. 'I write, do some teaching and research. I've resisted temptations to return to work, and I'm no longer involved in any discussion around mental health care in Orkney. That's finished.' I have mixed feelings about it. I wanted to be able to help but cannot provide what is really needed. Nevertheless, I remain in touch with some of the people trying to make a difference.

'I'm setting up a group of people to provide spiritual support to people who are sick . . . I wondered if you'd be interested? They will be supported themselves.'

I'm a little stunned. 'I'm not a religious person, at least not these days. I was once.'

'That doesn't matter, it's about being there for people, befriending them when they are coming to terms with what is happening to them in their lives.'

'So – "making sense" – what does it mean?' It sounds kind of familiar. Something like what I've been working through myself over the last couple of years. Trying to find some renewed meaning and purpose in life when your circumstances have changed, sometimes beyond recognition. Working out what is important to you and what you still want to do. I share my ideas with him, and he says, 'Yes, exactly that.'

'I'm not sure. It sounds like the kind of thing I might be able to do . . . can we talk about it when my situation here is a little clearer?'

I also don't know if I'm ready to on take something like that. However, having someone to fulfil that role can be so important when you are ill and trying to recover. Walking away from the building after saying goodbye and promising to think about it, I filed the Chaplain's suggestion away in my head to mull over on another day and discuss with John. It is so very hard to give up that desire of wanting to be useful when that has been your life, and if we do stay here in Orkney, I want to play an active part in this community to give something back. My friendships have been very important to me, but there are many people who aren't able to talk about painful topics with their loved ones or have no-one at all.

I have been listening to a long and searching interview I was invited to do for BBC Radio Orkney last January, talking about my experiences of both being a psychiatrist and experiencing depression. It has only recently been broadcast.

'We usually have a piece of music to play out the programme,' the interviewer told me. 'Maybe you'd like to think of something?'

I chose something from Brazil by João Gilberto, to introduce some welcome southern heat from the Brazilian summer into the Orkney winter, just for once. It also reminded me of the most important things in life: friendship and love.

One evening in Rio, almost two years ago, a cool breeze signalled a change in the weather and the risk of warm tropical showers. Sandra and I had waited until the last few of the red and black clad football fans from the Maracanã Stadium down the road had sauntered homewards, wrapped in the flag of their team *Flamengo*, before venturing to the bar down the road from her apartment. The place where she has lived all her life.

'How is the burger and beer?' she asked.

'The best I've had in a long time.' I waved to the barman for refills. 'It's been so good to see you.'

Sandra is one of the few people with whom I share the things that are really troubling me, especially the ones I am less proud of: wishing my mother-in-law ill, coping with that knowledge, living with the sense that our lives had been on hold because of her.

'I am worried about my family too,' she said.

Her two children, whom I first met as young teenagers, had grown into the adults we left behind at the apartment. Despite their problems, Sandra and her family have a profound sense of where they come from and who they are. She fights for her children with the zeal and courage of a lioness. I do not remember being the focus of such a powerful combination of maternal affection and ambition, but I do have the source of that energy as a friend.

Tonight, I can hear the storm raging behind the shutters we had fitted to keep out the sun in the white nights of summer. This small bedroom in Orkney sometimes feels like the cabin of a ship tossed in the high seas, but inside it feels safe, if not always so warm. I lie awake thinking about what I've written and trying to make sense of the recurring image of the snow globe from my journey back to childhood. As a child I was trapped and at the mercy of the violent storms within my family, yet also safely sealed off from the world. Perhaps I've always been ambivalent about my freedom, wanting to be both inside and outside that glass dome.

This evening, as I sat writing at my desk, John paused beside me. 'You really have impressed your personality on this house,' he said.

'What do you mean?'

'This room in particular. Your kitchen, the desk, your books...'

'And you have hung all the pictures properly, fixed the name sign outside and mended things when they break. I'm useless at anything practical. You had to rebuild the bed don't forget.' He managed to find a place for all the metal bits that I had left out. 'This is your home too...if you want it to be.'

One of his photographs hangs on the kitchen wall. An old black and white image that he took not very long after we first met, on our first journey north. It's not particularly flattering, but we've always liked it. The woman in it is standing at the door of a Hebridean cottage, arms folded in front of her with long hair blowing in the wind, scowling slightly at the camera, as always. It is me.

'You look very self-possessed. Holding your ground, like you just want to tell me to piss off.'

'Maybe I do, although I do look fairly relaxed about it.' I said, 'and we are still together.' Twenty-five years married this year.

I wonder how Katie the errant farm cat is getting on in her new home. Has she risked crossing the threshold or will she want to live in the barn forever? Has she overcome her ambivalence, and begun to enjoy the pleasures of domestication? Like her, I will probably always be semi-feral. However, weighing the alternatives on the scales of indecision, there are moments in life when we all need to consider not only what is best for us, but also for those we care deeply about.

I reach over to John, but he is asleep. So, I turn over again, trying to drop off again by focusing on my breath as it rhythmically warms the chill night air.

Unusually, the wind is light today. However, it's blowing from the North and bearing sleet. We are walking along the coastal path beyond Stromness, looking over the blue-black water to Hoy. The hills are shrouded in grey mist, but a watery sun is jostling its way between the clouds. Suddenly it emerges, casting an unworldly glow on the choppy waters of Scapa Flow.

'Do you remember that first time we came to Scotland together and we got caught out in the rain?'

'I left my coat in the car and we got the ferry to Iona?' He laughs. He had been certain that the day would be fair, but on islands the weather changes rapidly.

'Horizontal rain like you'd never known it.' We sat, soaked to the skin, he more than me as I had brought my waterproof, waiting for the ferry back to Mull, consoled by an extremely soggy dog who came over to us for affection.

'Just like here!' John is more cheerful than I have seen him for many months. Having grieved for his mother, he is beginning to look forward to the future.

'I'm so pleased I managed to spend those last couple of years with Mum,' he says as we walk back from the graveyard out by the coast near Warbeth. 'Taking her out, back to places that mattered to her.' Their old family home while she could still remember it.

Whilst looking in the huge mirror over the mantelpiece in the kitchen this morning, I was taken back to a moment long ago, before a similar mirror over a fireplace in my childhood home. I had been combing my hair and checking my makeup before going to the pub with my friends. Beyond my reflection, I could see my father standing behind me frowning as he watched me struggle to separate eyelashes stuck together with mascara.

'Do you want me to get out of the way?' I asked.

'No . . . just . . . I think you are going to manage fine, you know, in looks and in life.'

I don't remember my reply. Those times which can seem so important later, just pass inconsequentially in the moment. He had been trying to tell me that he still cared, to reassure me, only I didn't realise it then. It can take years, decades to remember the positive things about a relationship when it has been as complicated as it was between Dad and me, but I'm learning how to hold onto those memories whilst letting go of the painful ones.

Out at the Point of Ness we pause to watch for the seals that sometimes play there and gaze at the sky until the light begins to fade again. We have had a few days of respite from the gales though another storm is coming. We have just heard that we do have permission to extend the Wee Hoose and make it large enough for both of us, if we want to. We have a decision to make.

'Are you sure about this?' I ask John. 'Can you tolerate the winters on Orkney?'

'I am, yes, really.' He is getting excited about it. 'It will be a different house.'

'Yes, it will be larger, but it needs to be if we are to be here together.'

However, I know that if he didn't want to be here all the time, or if he decided that he couldn't cope with the wind and the rain, even though we have just had three marvellous days of cold winter sunshine, that would be fine too.

Our environment can play a crucial part in how we feel about life, but I am coming to see even more that true north isn't only a place, it is also a state of mind, and something that you hold within your heart. We all need to find a place that is the right fit for us. For you it may be a Pacific island or a room full of your family and friends, but what is most important is how being there enables us to nurture the strength growing inside us. Carrying the power of the image and sensations that go with it, until we can return. Navigating your way to that island is partly about having the courage to listen to your own 'distant drummer',[14] but it is also about acknowledging the importance of your relationships with other people, even if there is conflict between those different desires. Coming to terms with the contradictions is what life is about. I've been searching for my island of calm and sanity in the physical world, without realizing that it must inevitably occupy a space inside me too. Without it, no physical place will ever retain those qualities.

This morning the tree outside my desk window is silhouetted against a lighter sky as the fields beyond catch the rising sun. This is where I work and write. That will not change when the Wee Hoose is extended but there will also be space, with better light from a south facing window, to paint. The changing seasons and skies are my constant. Very soon the hares will run in the fields once again. They are there now, but they aren't ready to reveal themselves yet.

John places a cup of tea above my screen.

'I've been thinking about a couple of things . . . as I was writing.'

'Oh...'

'This would be a great place for a cat to sleep...' I point to the deep recess between my desk and the front window which would easily fit a cat bed.

'Hmm, good idea, although of course they choose their own place whatever you buy,' he muses, 'but if you put papers there you don't want them to sit on, they'll sit there anyway.' He knows there is more to come.

I take a deep breath. 'Do you think I might ever learn to swim? Would you teach me?' Trusting him more than anyone else to help me, I want to overcome the fear of water that I have had since childhood.

'It will probably end in divorce,' he laughs, giving me his hand.

'I won't let it,' I reply, holding it tight.

Across the valley a murmuration of starlings swoops and dives against the backdrop of a snow-capped Hoy.

Acknowledgements

People living with mental illness, especially my patients, taught me more about recovery than I could learn from lectures or books. The stories included here are all based on those of real people, but key details have been altered. The names of some others have also been changed.

Thanks to everyone who read earlier drafts including Wendy Burn, Tony Kendrick, André Tomlin, Kate Lovett, James Withey and especially Ruth Hunt. Thanks to the wonderful Jane Graham Maw at Graham Maw Christie, my editor Robert Davidson, Moira Forsyth and everyone at Sandstone Press. Thanks to all my friends, and everyone else who has kept me going, particularly Peter Talbot. Writing this book would not have been possible without the love and support of my husband, John Manton.

Notes

1. The sociologist Mike Bury called this the 'biographical disruption of chronic illness.'

2. Martin Buber the German philosopher distinguished between the attitude of 'I' towards 'it' – an object, and the attitude of 'I' towards 'Thou' in a living relationship.

3. Psychodynamic therapy is a form of talking therapy based on the ideas of Sigmund Freud. The impact of past relationships on the present is explored through the medium of the evolving relationship between the therapist and patient.

4. In cognitive therapy, the therapist asks you to identify the rules by which you live your life, which are often contradictory.

5. An experiment to test out strongly held beliefs which is used in cognitive behaviour therapy.

6. I have never been involved in trials of medication, but I have received funding for research assistants, speaking at meetings, travel and consultancy work for several major drug companies during my academic career.

7. Symptoms for which there is no clear medical cause, although if you look really hard you might find some physiological explanation for them, and sometimes, over time, the cause become clear. It's a controversial term as some patients think doctors are often too willing to blame everything on emotional problems, especially if you already have those too, which is 'diagnostic overshadowing'.

8. 'Hello my name is' was a campaign started by Kate Granger, a doctor who spent time having treatment for cancer before her untimely death. She noted how nobody ever introduced themselves in this way at the bedside.

9. I struggle with what sometimes has felt like the pseudo evangelical language of the 'recovery movement', a powerful group within the mental health community who have promoted a more 'positive' view of outcomes within mental health. This can have a negative impact on those who are struggling with hard realities. Beliefs or values cannot be imposed upon us by well-meaning priests or professionals.

10. Owen helped to found the co-operative movement, pioneered access to proper schooling for the children of New Lanark, and brought in a revolutionary eight-hour working day. He lived and died by his values of a com-

munal society in which people cared for each other, and those with money and influence, what we would now call privilege, had a responsibility to help those who did not.

11. The tentorium is a membrane just below the brain. Supratentorial means 'above' that, and in medical slang 'all in the head.'

12. Attachment theory emphasises the importance of a secure and trusting mother-infant bond on development and well-being.

13. A member of the Protestant Orange Order, most commonly associated with Northern Ireland, but also to be found in the Scottish Lowlands.

14. '*If a man does not keep pace with his companions, perhaps it is because he hears a different drummer. Let him step to the music which he hears, however measured or far away.*' This famous quotation from Thoreau's *Walden* was on the wall of my PhD supervisor's office. It always inspired.

Select bibliography

Bowring, J., *A Field Guide to Melancholy*. (Oldcastle Books, 2015)

Davies, W., *The happiness industry: How the government and big business sold us well-being*. (Verso Books, 2015)

Davidson, P., *The Idea of North*. (Reaktion Books, 2016)

Ehrenberg, A., *The weariness of the self: Diagnosing the history of depression in the contemporary age*. (McGill-Queen's Press-MQUP, 2016)

Ehrenreich, Barbara, *Smile or die: How positive thinking fooled America and the world*. (Granta Books, 2010)

Frank, A.W., *The wounded storyteller: Body, illness, and ethics*. (University of Chicago Press, 2013)

Frankl, V.E., *Man's search for meaning*. (Simon and Schuster, 1985)

Goldberg, D., Goodyer, I.M., *The origins and course of common mental disorders*. (Routledge, 2014)

Gilbert, P., *The Compassionate Mind: A New Approach to Life's Challenges.* (Constable-Robinson, 2009)

Holloway, R., *On forgiveness: How can we forgive the unforgivable?* (Canongate Books, 2002)

van der Kolk, B., *The body keeps the score.* (New York: Viking, 2014)

Kramer, P.D., *Ordinarily well: the case for antidepressants.* Farrar, (Straus and Giroux, 2016)

Mabey, R., *Nature cure.* (Random House, 2011)

Miller, A., *The drama of the gifted child: The search for the true self.* (Basic Books, 2008)

Moran, J., *Shrinking Violets: The Secret Life of Shyness.* (Profile Books, 2016)

Phillips, A., and B. Taylor, *On kindness.* (Macmillan, 2009)

Pilgrim, D., and A. McCranie, *Recovery and mental health: A critical sociological account.* (Macmillan, 2013)

Ridge, D., *Recovery from depression using the narrative approach.* (Jessica Kingsley Publishers, 2009)

Rufus, A., *Party of One: the loner's manifesto.* (Avalon, 2008)

Ryle, A., & I.B. Kerr, *Introducing cognitive analytic therapy: Principles and practice.* (John Wiley & Sons, 2003)

Slingerland, E.G., *Trying Not to Try: Ancient China, Modern Science, and the Power of Spontaneity.* (Broadway Books, 2015)

Solomon, A., *The Noonday Demon: An atlas of depression.* (Simon and Schuster, 2001)

Storr, A., *Solitude: A return to the self.* (Simon and Schuster, 2005)

Weisbrode, K., *On ambivalence: the problems and pleasures of having it both ways.* (MIT Press, 2012)

Yalom, I.D., *Existential psychotherapy* (Vol. 1) (Basic books, 1980)